Master Your Mind and Energy to Heal Your Body

You can be your own cure

Brandy Gillmore

Foreword by David Perlmutter, M.D.

WELBECK
BALANCE

Published in 2024 by Welbeck Balance
An imprint of Welbeck Non-Fiction Limited
Part of Welbeck Publishing Group
Offices in: London – 20 Mortimer Street, London W1T 3JW &
Sydney – Level 17, 207 Kent St, Sydney NSW 2000 Australia
www.welbeckpublishing.com
Design and layout © Welbeck Non-Fiction Ltd 2024
Text © Brandy Gillmore 2024

ISBN
978-1-80129-221-4

Typeset by Lapiz Digital Services
Printed in Great Britain by Clays Ltd, Elcograf S.p.A.

10 9 8 7 6 5 4 3 2

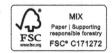

Author's Note

While the stories of healing in this book involve real people, names and details have been changed to protect the privacy of those involved as well as that of their families. If there is resemblance to any person, it is purely coincidental. In some places, the timeline of events and information may also be modified to provide the reader with step-by-step clarity or to include newer research. The author of this book does not diagnose, treat, dispense medical advice, nor prescribe the use of any technique as a form of treatment for emotional, physical, medical, or mental illness directly or indirectly. The intention of this book is solely to provide helpful and informative material of a general nature to help support your journey for emotional and spiritual well-being. If you do use any of the information in this book, then it is advised to do so only under the care of a physician or appropriate licensed professional. The author, publisher, and all affiliates disclaim all responsibility for any liability arising directly or indirectly from the use or misuse of the information contained in this book.

Publisher's Note/Disclaimer

Welbeck encourages and welcomes diversity and different viewpoints. However, all views, thoughts, and opinions expressed in this book are the author's own and are not necessarily representative of Welbeck Publishing Group as an organization. Welbeck Publishing Group makes no representations or warranties of any kind, express or implied, with respect to the accuracy, completeness, suitability or currency of the contents of this book, and specifically disclaims, to the extent permitted by law, any implied warranties of merchantability or fitness for a particular purpose and any injury, illness, damage, death, liability or loss incurred, directly or indirectly from the use or application of any of the information contained in this book. This book is intended for informational purposes and guidance only, and is not intended to replace, diagnose, treat or act as a substitute for professional, expert medical and/or psychiatric advice. The author and the publisher are not medical practitioners nor counsellors, and professional advice should be sought before embarking on any health-related program. Any names, characters, trademarks, service marks and trade names detailed in this book are the property of their respective owners and are used solely for identification and reference purposes. This book is a publication of Welbeck Non-Fiction, part of Welbeck Publishing Group and has not been licensed, approved, sponsored or endorsed by any person or entity. Every reasonable effort has been made to trace copyright holders of material produced in this book, but if any have been inadvertently overlooked the publishers would be glad to hear from them.

ENDORSEMENTS

"When I met Brandy Gillmore, it was to conduct a case study at Psy-Tek Lab to demonstrate the mind's ability to relieve physical pain. During our collaboration, I observed Brandy guiding participants on how to use their own minds. Brandy's approach was unlike anything I had seen before. As each person utilized their own mind, they reported a significant reduction or even complete elimination of their physical pain. Simultaneously, I was able to document physiological changes taking place in the body using medical thermal imaging. It was also remarkable that several participants had already tried mindfulness and positive thinking practices prior to the study, which had not resolved their chronic pain. After witnessing Brandy's method, I firmly believe that everyone should learn how to utilize this innovative approach to working with their minds. I am pleased that Brandy has decided to write a book to share her method. I am convinced that it will contribute to the dissemination of this innovative method of working with the mind, which is most needed in our present world."

Gaetan Chevalier, Ph.D. Director of Research at Psy-Tek Labs, Lead Faculty at the California Institute of Human Sciences, Visiting Scholar in the Department of Family Medicine and Public Health at UCSD

"Having worked with Brandy, not only over the years but recently through COVID-19, I've been able to focus and release stored toxic energy and traumatic ideas. I highly recommend this work. It's centering, balancing, healing, and moreover, self-empowering."

Sharon Stone, Actor, Producer and Artist

"I highly recommend this book. It is empowering and has the ability to transform the way the world sees health and healing."

Jack Canfield, Co-author of the *Chicken Soup for the Soul®* series and *The Success Principles ™*

"In *Master Your Mind and Energy to Heal Your Body*, Brandy Gillmore provides a valuable perspective on the ability to promote healing, along with a wide range of tools and techniques for enhancing physical recovery through the mind-body connection. A must read."

Anita Moorjani, New York Times Best-selling Author of *Dying To Be Me*, *What if this is Heaven* and *Sensitive is the New Strong*

"Brandy Gillmore's book offers a revolutionary perspective on the power of the mind and the ability we each hold to heal ourselves. I wholeheartedly recommend it."

Barnet Bain, Film Producer on *What Dreams May Come*

"I was profoundly moved by Brandy's remarkable story. This book is not only beautifully written but also incredibly inspiring. Understanding the power of Brandy's own transformation gives me great hope for those suffering with physical pain. This book is an absolute must-read!"

Katherine Woodward Thomas, *New York Times* Best-selling Author of *Calling in "The One"* and *Conscious Uncoupling*

"How does one explain the miraculous? In this powerful book, Brandy Gillmore does just that as she takes your hand and walks you, step by step, out of the world of chronic suffering into a new and pain-free life. Using her personal experience, with massive amounts of supporting science and data, you truly can *Master Your Mind and Energy to Heal Your Body* (and become your own cure)."

Arielle Ford, Author of *The Love Thief*

"I love Brandy's book! I love the way she has skillfully and caringly woven her successful healing story, her extraordinary research, and her wonderful practice into healing and empowerment for everyone who reads it. If you want to unlock your innate healing power, I highly recommend reading Brandy's book. You will be inspired, as am I, to use Brandy's method, which opens up new pathways for your self-healing and freedom to live a happy life."

Dr. Anita Sanchez, Trainer and Author of International Award-winning *The Four Sacred Gifts: Indigenous Wisdom for Modern Times*

"The doctoral training I attended to become a Psychotherapist was in a traditional setting. There was really no talk, training or focus on the power of the mind, body, and spirit to impact general well-being. Furthermore, the focus was on pathology, versus the innate strength we have as human beings to heal and prevail. In this "gift" of a book, author Brandy Gillmore offers a perspective that embraces all of these dimensions of who we are. She takes us beyond the theory of illness, into the healing power we all have within… providing us with effective tools to heal what is ailing us and live in a state of feeling GOOD.

From her personal experience of overcoming serious physiological obstacles, Brandy embodies the knowing and expertise to lead us to a better tomorrow, leaving us confident in her knowledge and guidance and in our own journey to create and receive optimal physical, mental, and emotional health. Most of us have, are, or will face some kind of medical challenge. This book belongs right on our bedside and will be the best "get better" book you can gift someone you care about. Bravo Brandy and thank you for this GIFT!"

Marcy Cole, Ph.D.

"Since the day I met Brandy and heard her story of miraculous healing, I've been a super fan. But I had no idea the power she possessed in helping others—including me—to heal themselves. There is not merely "theory" here. To experience Brandy's work, directly or in this book, is to be met with a soul force that can't be denied—and won't let you deny yourself! I mean this in the best way, that she is unrelenting in her commitment and capacity to help you heal and become liberated from the unconscious patterns that sabotage us all. I've worked with and known many of the biggest healers and teachers in the 20 years I've been in the field of self-help, and Brandy is one of the best-kept secrets (but not for long). More than her GIFT method, Brandy is the gift that keeps on giving! Don't just read this book; soak it up, be in her presence, and prepare for your own miracle."

Derek Rydall, Author of *Emergence: Seven Steps for Radical Life Change* and *The Abundance Project: 40 Days to More Wealth, Health, Love and Happiness*

"I have seen the miracles that Brandy Gillmore has produced for people desperate to get out of physical and emotional pain, but not until I read her book, *Master Your Mind and Energy to Heal Your Body*, did I finally understand exactly how she guided people to their own life-changing miracles. This book makes it so clear! It's also a fascinating read about how she put these pieces together with her insatiable passion and brilliant research-mind in search of a cure for her own terrible suffering. Let's all follow Brandy's genius to our own healing!"

Jackie Lapin, Author of Two International Best-sellers and Founder of SpeakerTunity®—The Speaker & Leader Research Company

"I've had the privilege of hosting Brandy on my show numerous times. Her work is inspiring, shedding light on the path to genuine healing. I've witnessed her empower individuals by teaching them how to use their own minds to release emotional and physical pain. In this book, Brandy shares the invaluable insights behind her innovative process.

She also shares her incredible personal journey, compelling case studies, and a revolutionary perspective that can help bridge the gap between Western medicine and miraculous healing. Her book is a powerful tool for anyone seeking to heal their mind and body, and it serves as a testament to the incredible potential of the human spirit."

John Burgos, Producer and Host on *Beyond The Ordinary* show

"I am excited for anyone who has found their way to this book, especially if you have tried everything to heal, manifest, or improve your life in order to feel happy and whole. In *Master Your Mind and Energy to Heal Your Body*, Brandy Gillmore provides an easy-to-follow, step-by-step roadmap to optimal health. Using your thoughts, emotions, and actions, you can shift your energy to heal yourself and transcend your emotional and physical pain from the past, allowing you to thrive as the best version of yourself. I highly recommend this book!"

Natalie Ledwell, Best-selling Author and Co-founder of MindMovies.com

"Thank you, Brandy, for your loving contribution to my own personal healing in ways too numerous to mention. And thank you for so masterfully sharing your incredible journey and then generously giving us the GIFT of your 4-step healing modality. The moment in Chapter 1 when you had your epiphany about placebos gave me goosebumps from head to toe. This book is a miracle and a must-read for anyone who wants to know the truth about how to live with radiant health."

Debra Poneman, Best-selling Author and Founder of Yes to Success, Inc.

"Over the past several years, I have watched Brandy show people how to access the power of the mind to release pain within minutes! I experienced this for myself as well. Our minds are powerful. This book that Brandy has written is much needed for our time. She masterfully bridges science and spirituality to show the intricate link between mind and body. Her ideas are revolutionary; this book gives individuals the power to heal their lives by using techniques that are easy to incorporate into daily life. Reading it, I felt like I was sitting down talking to a mentor or friend. The writing is accessible and knowledgeable. It's a life-changing read!"

Rachel Lang, author of *Modern Day Magic: 8 Simple Rules to Realize Your Power and Shape Your Life*

"If you have invested countless time and energy into changing your life, especially your health, and it just doesn't seem to be changing, this book is the answer to your prayers. Brandy's GIFT method walks you through how to empower yourself to actually heal—for good! Her compassion combined with scientific backing is just the recipe we all need to take our lives back into our own hands with the power of our minds."

Christine Hassler, Author, Podcast Host and Master Coach

"Brandy embodies what it really means to utilize the full healing power of the mind and she is on a mission to help people realize our own potential. Brandy's passion and enthusiasm for what is possible is contagious and her brilliant insights spark the truth that can set you free. I am grateful she is able to clearly explain a process in her book we can use to live up to our full potential. Follow every word!"

Lisa Garr, host of *The Aware Show*

FOREWORD

In the ever-evolving field of medicine, where the mysteries of the human body are ceaselessly explored, we often lean heavily on tangible and quantifiable solutions. My journey as a physician and specifically as a neurologist has been steeped in this physical, data-driven approach, at least until the later stages of my career. The accepted dogma in mainstream medicine is that a pill, a procedure, or a regimen is the hallmark of addressing human suffering, particularly when it comes to pain. However, every so often, a voice emerges that challenges the status quo and beckons us to peer beyond the traditional. Brandy Gillmore's *Master Your Mind and Energy to Heal Your Body* is one such clarion call, lovingly inviting us to look deeper, where the mind meets matter.

Brandy's narrative is a testament, woven from the fabric of personal struggle and enlightenment. The pain that she encountered following an accident was debilitating and unrelenting. But what sets Brandy's experience apart is not the nature of her suffering, but her audacious response to it. While many would resign to their fate or remain dependent on the palliative effects of medicine, she embarked on an odyssey within, navigating the intricate labyrinth of her mind.

In this book, Brandy brilliantly elucidates the profound interplay between our thoughts, our energy, and our physical health. She postulates, with compelling conviction, that harnessing the power of the mind can be an instrumental force in healing. This isn't to diminish the merits of medical interventions; rather, it's an invitation to expand our armamentarium, to include tools that reside *within each of us*, often untapped and unacknowledged.

Calling it like it is, the tenets that Brandy espouses have long been overlooked in conventional medical curricula. I confess, as I delved into the early pages, I too grappled with the duality of my training and the transformative insights Brandy presented. But as I journeyed with her, what unfurled was not a repudiation of my medical education but an augmentation of it. Medicine and mind, as Brandy showcases, aren't antithetical but synergistic.

The methodology that Brandy shares is steeped in the principle of positive embodiment. It's a radical shift from the passive receipt of care to an *active engagement* in one's healing process. This involves a deliberate reprogramming, a cleansing of the negative thoughts and energies that often tether us to our ailments. Brandy doesn't just preach these concepts; she's a living testament to their efficacy.

It's an undeniable truth that our mental state, our beliefs, and our energies profoundly impact our health. Be it the placebo effect or the adverse outcomes seen in patients with chronic stress or depression, the mind's role in health is irrefutable. And yet, ironically, this potent ally often remains sidelined in our treatment strategies. Brandy's work rectifies this oversight, offering a roadmap to enlist the mind as a formidable partner in our healing journey.

What resonates profoundly is the universality of Brandy's teachings. Whether one is ensnared in the throes of chronic pain, as she once was, or battling other health challenges, the techniques she delineates are universally applicable. They serve as a beacon, not just for patients but for healthcare providers, urging us to broaden our perspectives and integrate mind mastery into our therapeutic approaches.

This is essential reading for both those receiving care as well as those who provide it. And for the latter, this book fills the gaps that our education might have inadvertently overlooked. It's an invitation to integrate care, in a way that mind and body aren't disparate entities but a cohesive unit, each influencing the other.

Brandy Gillmore's work is a clarion call to look within, to tap into the latent power of our minds, and to harness this force for our well-being.

David Perlmutter, M.D.
October, 2023
Naples, Florida, USA

CONTENTS

INTRODUCTION

What if I told you that the power to heal yourself is not found in some expensive new treatment, but instead in the power of your own mind? Further, what if I told you it's become my new norm to see people heal themselves from a variety of health issues they were told were incurable?

Given that you've picked up this book, it's likely you've heard that our minds are incredible and possess the power to heal. After all, the concept of healing through thoughts, emotions, or prayers has been documented for thousands of years in nearly every spiritual teaching—from Buddhism, Catholicism, and Christian Science to New Age spiritual practices. There's even a branch of traditional Western medicine called psychoneuroimmunology, which examines the complex interplay between psychological factors, the nervous system, and the immune system, including how our minds can impair our immune system and affect our health. However, using the power of the mind to heal is not an area that human beings have truly mastered.

Sadly, despite trillions of dollars being spent on healthcare each year on the billions of people around the world impacted by chronic pain and illness, the number of people suffering is not decreasing; instead, the numbers are increasing. We must be willing to expand our approach—and I can show you how.

Could you imagine a world in which we have all learned to master our own minds to heal ourselves?

In the pages that follow, I will share with you the same insights, tools and techniques that I have shared with others to help them heal themselves from a myriad of issues they were told were incurable. This includes everything from chronic pain and years of migraines to autoimmune conditions, being bedridden, depression, anxiety, and everything in between. As you will see in the coming pages, our bodies really do have an incredible, innate ability to heal themselves.

If you're living with chronic pain or illness, like so many people, likely you have also heard the common words: "There's nothing more we can do for you." "This is a condition that you'll have to deal with for the rest of your life." "I'll prescribe you something for the pain."

You may have tried numerous healing remedies and approaches—from traditional treatments, diets, exercise, and supplements, to practices like mindfulness, visualization, positive thinking, affirmations, gratitude practices, and various alternative therapies.

I know firsthand from my work helping thousands of people to heal themselves that many people have either known about the power of the mind to heal but have been unable to get any real results for themselves, and/or found the idea of the mind healing the body unrealistic, or "too good to be true."

Personally, I experienced both of these things.

In 2003, my world changed in an instant when an accident rendered me disabled and in excruciating pain. My pain was so deep that it hurt to breathe and hurt to move. I saw some of the best doctors and specialists, and no matter how skilled and wonderful my doctors were, my body was not healing. It was not their fault; there was nothing any of them could do.

Desperate for relief, I tried everything from nerve ablations, infusions, and injections, to diets, supplements, and practices like visualization, positive thinking, affirmations, and various alternative practices. While some things could decrease my pain at times, they didn't heal my body. Part of me wanted to give up, but I knew I couldn't spend the rest of my life in excruciating pain.

Initially, the idea of using my mind to heal my physical body seemed nonsensical to me. However, after years of research into medically documented phenomena, I made some eye-opening discoveries.

It's important to note that when some people hear the term "healing with the mind," they mistakenly believe it means the problems are "all in your head," or using "mind over matter," but this isn't the case at all. Instead, using the power of the mind to heal the body starts with the foundational awareness that every part of your physical body is connected to, and controlled by, your brain. We can see evidence of this mind-body connection when a person suffers a brain injury or a stroke, resulting in physical impairment or paralysis.

As I reflected on this well-known awareness of the mind-body connection during my own healing exploration, I began to ask myself: *If the brain is directly connected to every part of our body, and has the power to control every part of the body, then wouldn't it make sense that it also possesses the influence to heal every part of the body too?*

This ultimately led me to start my own detailed research into the topic of healing, which I'll be sharing with you in Part One of this book. After six years of researching, including lots of experimentation on myself, I finally was able to make an incredible breakthrough and discovered exactly what I needed to do to completely heal myself. As a result, I was able to make a *full* recovery using only the power of my mind. That was back in 2010. Since then, I'm delighted to say that I've remained 100 percent pain-free and healthy.

After my recovery, people around me asked how they could heal themselves. Like me, they were suffering and often felt hopeless. Soon, they were able to heal themselves, using the same process I created for myself. At that point, instead of going back into my previous line of work in the field of technology, I wanted to find effective ways to share what I had discovered about the power of our mind to heal our body with as many people as possible.

Since there was no traditional certification or school for the healing insights I had discovered, I decided to get qualified in a range of healing approaches—from alternative schools and universities that taught spiritual counseling, quantum healing, and everything in between. Then I set out to help others.

For many people, the idea of healing with the mind may sound impossible. For that reason, I began searching for a way to demonstrate mind-body healing with medical equipment. In 2015, I was able to demonstrate mind-body healing for the first time, live, using medical thermal imaging. People could literally see the power of their minds with their own eyes. This is something that has never been done before. I will share more details with you in the coming pages.

Since my recovery, I've had the honor of working with thousands of people around the world to help them heal— through a combination of courses, classes, and workshops, both in person and online. My clients have included people from all walks of life and all ages battling various health issues, including people who have spent most of their lives sick and in pain, as well as people with recent health problems, and everything in between.

My hope in writing this book is to help as many people as possible learn to use their incredible self-healing ability.

I've seen time and time again that once people have been able to understand the GIFT Mind-Body Healing approach to working with their mind, they have been able to get tangible results—even those who had previously spent years looking for solutions and trying any modality they could find without success.

Much like we are born with an ability to learn to read and write, the same is true with healing; we have an innate ability to heal ourselves, but it's a skill that we must first learn to do. In Part One, I will reveal the hidden research and groundbreaking discoveries that helped me understand our ability to heal ourselves.

Then in Part Two, I will share with you the step-by-step process I call the GIFT Method. As the name alludes, this process was a life-changing gift. This is because as you reprogram your mind for healing, you can also simultaneously change your life. I have worked with thousands of people who have been able to improve everything from their health to their levels of energy, happiness, love, relationships, and personal fulfillment.

During the depths of my suffering, if someone had told me that my illness and injury would ultimately lead me to a life-changing gift, I would have had a hard time conceiving that this was possible. However, to my surprise, once I began to reprogram and master my mind, it really did happen.

It has now become my norm to see people heal themselves from all types of health issues using the methods that I share with you in this book. I receive messages from people all of the time, telling me how shocked their doctors are that they have been able to heal from an "incurable" pain or illness. I've had people's parents, partners, and other family members reach out to thank me because their loved one is now healed and has their life back. Of course, I tell them that it wasn't me who did it; each individual has been able to use the insights and techniques of the GIFT Method to heal themselves. I'll share the stories of some of these people in the pages ahead in the hope that you, too, will be able to use the same insights and techniques to change your health and your life. In short, the steps of the GIFT Method are:

- **Step G: Get** new healthy mind programming
- **Step I: Identify** the specific problems that can block your healing and affect your health
- **Step F: Free Yourself** from negative emotional energy and miswired mind programming that is connected to your illness
- **Step T: Transform** yourself by reprogramming and releasing unhealthy mind programming and then embody the transformation to get lasting results

Each step builds on the previous one, which means that it's best to go through the book in order.

Within each of these steps, you will find a range of simple but incredibly powerful tools and techniques that will empower you to change your mindset and connect with your body's innate ability to heal.

Regardless of where you are with your health right now, healing with your mind really can work for you. The key is learning how to *master* your mind.

Note: It is common for me to see people have such great results that they no longer need their medication. However, keep in mind that, per the law, *only* your doctor or licensed professional can make changes to your prescription or medical treatment plan. For that reason, when you implement the process, you'll want to remain under the care of your doctor and let them know what you are doing so they can continue to monitor your health and any medications you are taking.

Whether you've been suffering from pain or illness for a long time or it's a recent development, I feel genuine compassion for you as well as genuine excitement that you will soon know how to harness the strength, energy, and self-healing power within your own mind to heal your body and live the healthy, happy life you truly deserve.

Ready? Let's get started.

PART ONE

INCURABLE TO CURED

The Research That Helped Me Heal Myself and How It Can Help You Heal Yourself

1

THE INJURY THAT OPENED MY EYES TO SELF-HEALING

The most common way people give up their power is by thinking they don't have any.

—Alice Walker[1]

I didn't see it coming.

The accident, the injury, and the excruciating pain.

Before that fateful event, I had never envisioned myself using a wheelchair, walker, or cane to get around. And it never occurred to me that one day, doctors would tell me there was nothing further they could do for me.

Based on the way my life had been going, this turn of events was the last thing I expected. Growing up, I had been physically fit and had won several gold medals in martial arts at the Junior Olympics. I excelled in school and started college early. Eager to get out into the world, I began a career in technology where I worked for some of the largest telecommunications companies as a network operations technician and a network data test engineer. I had a passion for the world of technology; it was new, fast-paced, and exciting. I was quickly making my way up the corporate ladder, and it was perfect timing—the dot.com era was booming. My specialty was finding solutions to seemingly impossible network problems—I received recognition from several companies in the industry and then wrote a manual to help train others on how to do this.

Life was good. I had a great career, my own house, a caring romantic relationship, and wonderful friends and family. My days were full with never a dull moment.

THE ACCIDENT

My last "normal" day began on a happy note. My father's birthday celebration was coming up, and because he had always done so much for me, I wanted to do something special for him. After shopping and finding the perfect gift, I headed for home just as it started to sprinkle. Soon the drizzle turned into a downpour, and the rain was coming down so hard it sounded like the car was being pummeled with gravel.

My house was still thirty minutes away and traffic had begun to back up. I was thirsty and wanted a break from driving in the rain, so I found a convenience store to make a quick stop. As I walked toward the counter to buy a bottle of water, I slipped and crashed on the wet tile floor. The sound of the impact was so loud that both the customers and the staff turned to see what was going on and then immediately rushed over to help. Trying to catch my breath, I lay there, not moving, gasping as excruciating pain ripped through my back and down my legs. A woman made her way through the circle of people surrounding me and knelt down beside me.

"I'm a nurse," she said. "Don't move. Lie perfectly still." She turned toward the gathering crowd and yelled, "Someone call an ambulance!"

"I'm okay," I insisted, trying to keep calm. The last thing I wanted to do was be taken to the hospital. Having practiced martial arts for years, I had experienced injuries and was used to pushing through pain. I tried to reassure myself that I just needed to stand up and walk it off. But I couldn't. Each time I tried to get up, the pain shot more intensely through my body.

"Don't move," she repeated. "We need to be sure you haven't broken your neck."

She kept insisting that I be taken to the hospital. But I hated hospitals. And I was pretty sure the doctors would likely say that I had exacerbated an old back injury from a car accident a few years prior and then send me home with pain meds. From my previous injuries, I knew the ropes. I didn't want to waste the whole day in hospital, nor did I want any pain meds.

Even though moving caused intense pain, all I wanted to do was to escape the crowd of strangers huddled around me, waiting to see if I could get up. Knowing that I needed to do something, I lifted my head off the ground and turned it from side to side to show them my neck was fine. I told the nurse I would be okay with just a little time, but inwardly I knew this pain was worse than anything I'd ever felt. I think I was trying to convince myself more than her that I would be okay.

After a while, I persuaded the nurse that if she would just help me to my car to lie down, I would call my doctor from there. After a few people helped shoulder me to the car, I kept my word. Since it was the weekend, an on-call physician returned my call, and his words echoed those of the off-duty nurse: "You really need to go to the hospital."

Assuming the most they'd do was give me pain meds, I didn't heed his advice. Instead, I asked a friend to drive me home where I spent the rest of the day and night in extreme pain and unable to sleep. The next day was worse. The more I tried to move around, the less I could do.

SEARCHING FOR A CURE

The following day I relented and made an appointment to see my doctor. After the standard examinations and X-rays, he told me I had reinjured the same part of my back that had been damaged in the car accident, making it significantly worse, and there were some other injuries too. He prescribed pain medications and advised me to rest and move as little as possible.

Still, I tried to push through. However, instead of experiencing the improvement I had hoped for, the debilitating pain became more intense and began to burn. I had to take what I thought would be a short leave of absence from work and assured my colleagues that I would return soon.

At this point, my doctor referred me to a specialist. And when that specialist couldn't help me, I moved on to another, and then another. Each one tried different procedures and medications, but nothing worked. I traveled to the best hospitals and saw top consultants, but everyone was stumped on how to help me.

Most of my days were spent in bed, propped up on pillows, suffering not only extreme pain but growing depression. I was missing out on life. I did what I could when I could, and some days were worse than others. On a good day, I pushed through the pain. My doctors had given me a walker and cane for shorter distances and a wheelchair for longer distances, so I was able to get around on my own. But on a bad day, I couldn't make it out of bed.

Prescription pain medications, including morphine sulfate, barely took the edge off. When my doctors increased my dosage of morphine, I felt tired and "out of it." I didn't like that feeling, so I chose the lower dose and lived in nonstop pain.

I was broken in every sense of the word: physically, emotionally, and mentally. As the months went by, my health continued to decline to the point that I barely recognized myself. The outgoing, confident, and active woman I'd once been was gone, replaced with a shell of who I was. I went from feeling excited about my life to hitting rock bottom, living in fear, and not knowing what to do. My employer had been kind enough to hold my position open for much longer than was required by law, but eventually they had to hire a replacement.

Desperate, I continued to search for answers. With each specialist there were new tests, new procedures, and new medications. I was advised that I had a long list of ailments: nerve lesions, spondylosis, sciatica, spinal end-plate fractures, synovial cysts in my lumbar spine, and complex regional pain syndrome (CRPS). Having never heard of CRPS before, I began to research it. And the more I read, the more I didn't want to know—but I forced myself to keep reading.

CRPS, defined by the Stanford School of Medicine, is "a severely disabling condition that usually affects the limbs after injury or surgery. The main symptoms are severe pain, swelling, loss of range of motion, temperature changes, and changes in the skin. The degree of pain is severe and is usually much greater than the injury would typically cause."[2]

Many experts classify CRPS with nerve lesions as the most painful chronic pain condition known.[3] As a result, many CRPS sufferers fall into a state of hopelessness and are considered a high risk for suicide.[4]

I certainly knew the feeling. I was in extreme pain and found myself falling in and out of states of hopelessness. I had to do something, so I began searching for any solutions or shred of hope I could find. On the days I didn't do any research, my mind went to a dark place and my thoughts scared me. It became apparent that I couldn't allow myself to stop looking for answers. As a result, research became both an addiction and a form of emotional survival.

Despite my efforts, my health continued to decline. The longer I was immobile, the more pain I felt, and the more my muscles atrophied from limited use. As a result, I became very weak and developed osteopenia (reduced bone density) from lack of weight-bearing movement. It was a horrific cycle and I was a mess.

Doctors continued to do everything they could think of to lessen the pain: injections, nerve ablations, infusions, and arthroscopic procedures. But nothing provided any lasting relief.

I tried to remain hopeful, but each specialist gave me that same somber look and said something like, "I'm sorry, Ms. Gillmore, but there's nothing else I can do for you."

Every time I heard those words, my heart sank. With a lump in my throat, I'd hold back tears and collect my voice enough to ask for a referral for somebody else... anybody else. I begged until they came up with a new referral because I couldn't bear to leave their office without having at least some small hope that I would get better.

Most nights I was unable to sleep for more than a few hours before the pain pierced me awake. One day faded into the next. I spent a lot of time counting down the days—and sometimes hours—until I saw the next specialist, hoping he or she would be "the one" to change it all and help me get my life back.

Due to the heavy medications I was on, refills required in-person visits. I'd sit in the waiting rooms in my wheelchair and sometimes strike up conversations with others to see what treatments they were exploring. Some seemed resigned to their conditions, while others, like me, were exhausted but still held a glimmer of hope. Unfortunately, solutions seemed elusive.

I began to look at the American healthcare system and saw that it wasn't nearly as effective as I had previously thought. And it wasn't just me who wasn't healing. The more I researched, the more I learned just how many people were sick and in pain. Some reports showed as many as 70 percent of all Americans were taking at least one prescription medication.[5] And this kind of dire situation wasn't just in the United States; chronic illness was also rapidly increasing in most other countries around the world.[6-10]

I wondered if it might be because people were living longer, but I noted that illness wasn't just increasing in the elderly population. Statistics showed that illness was increasing in people of every age, including children.

It was alarming, to say the least, that despite all the advances in healthcare and technology, our collective health seemed to be getting worse. I continued to struggle to get through each day. I had wonderful, loving people who were there for me, and I was grateful for them—family and friends who helped me as much as they could, who did more than I could have ever asked for. But there was nothing they could do to help me get my life back.

I tried everything, including a deep dive into healing diets, nutritional supplements, acupuncture, reflexology, chiropractic, various types of meditation, positive thinking, visualization, and every modality I could think of. I refused to give up.

THE MEDICAL TRIAL

Through an unexpected turn of events, one of the hospitals in which I had been receiving treatments called to notify me that I was eligible to join a study that could help treat my chronic pain. Excited, I began counting down the days. My mind was filled with all the things I would do when I was healed—the places I would go and the friends I would visit. I smiled for the first time in weeks.

Finally, the day arrived. At the hospital a nurse wheeled me into a private curtained space and then helped me out of my wheelchair and onto the gurney. With growing anticipation, I watched as she hooked me up to machines that would monitor my vitals.

It's really happening.

Since this was a clinical trial, I knew it was going to be a double-blind study, which meant that half of the participants would receive the new injections while the other half would receive the placebo. If you're not familiar with a placebo, it's a fake treatment (e.g., a sugar pill) that is supposed to have no therapeutic value. Placebos are used in medical studies to assess the effectiveness of new drugs or treatments. They serve as a benchmark for comparing the outcomes against actual treatment. I prayed that I would get the *real* treatment and not the placebo.

As the doctor approached, the grim look on his face told me that something was wrong.

"Ms. Gillmore, I've reviewed your chart and your physical condition, and I would really like to help you, but I'm sorry. You can't be a part of this study." I felt a lump in my throat and my heart sank to the floor as he looked down at his clipboard and said the words I'll never forget. "We don't expect it to help you."

Devastated, I begged him to let me try.

"I wish I could," he said with a look of compassion. "But we can't afford to skew the results of the study by including patients who are unlikely to benefit from it."

Unlikely to benefit. I felt my eyes welling up with tears and I pleaded with him until he left the room. *It must be some kind of mistake.* But then the nurse solemnly began to unhook me from the machines and helped me change back into my clothes. She didn't utter a word. It was clear she didn't know what to say.

As she helped me back into my wheelchair, I focused on trying not to fall apart.

Suddenly, the doctor returned. To my surprise, he informed me that he had consulted the other researchers and, since the medication had already undergone extensive testing to prove that it was safe, he had been given approval to administer a round of the injections to me. However, he made it clear that my results would have to be kept separate from the official study.

After an emotional roller coaster, things were looking up! I didn't care if I was part of the official study or not. I just wanted to heal. I felt a surge of relief and anticipation as he gave me the injections with hopes they would give me my life back.

I don't remember the ride home, but when I woke up, I felt disoriented. The relentless pain was still burning and radiating throughout my body. Memories came flooding back of the trip to the hospital—the doctor, the upset, the sudden hope, and the injections.

I lay there awake but didn't even want to open my eyes. My head spun with disappointment and defeat. The doctor was right. The treatment that I believed, hoped, and prayed would give me back my life hadn't worked.

Suddenly, the spiraling thoughts stopped and a single clear thought came into my mind: *What about the placebo?* It was something I hadn't even considered. But as I thought about the studies in general, a certain percentage of people got some type of results from the placebo alone. I found myself wondering how the placebo effect works and if it was possible to intentionally activate it.

If the answer was yes, could I somehow use this information to heal myself? Curious and out of options, I began to explore this phenomenon in more depth.

2

IT TAKES MORE THAN JUST BELIEF TO HEAL

Nothing in life is to be feared, it is only to be understood. Now is the time to understand more, so that we may fear less.

—Marie Curie[1]

As I lay in bed searching for hope, I thought about the lead-up to the medical trial. I remembered thinking to myself hundreds of times over: *Please don't give me the placebo. I want the real treatment.*

But now I started to think about this differently.

After all, in many studies, a percentage of the participants who take the placebo experience improvements in their physical health as if they had taken the real medicine. Participants can experience measurable changes in their blood pressure, levels of pain, depression, IBS symptoms, sleep disorders, menopause issues, and many other conditions, including marked improvement in Parkinson's disease.[2-8]

I couldn't stop thinking about it. I knew it was not the full answer to my health because research had shown that the placebo does not typically result in a complete and lasting healing. However, the mere fact that it could work meant that it was *proven* that the mind has the ability to influence the physical body.[9] I wondered what mechanism in the mind caused the placebo to work, and if I could somehow activate it to heal my body.

I reviewed every study I could find—not just the positive results but also the negative ones. Negative results can occur when participants are given what they think is a treatment and are told there can be negative side effects. Such purported negative side effects are referred to as the "nocebo effect"—a term coined by Walter Kennedy back in 1961.[10]

One study conducted by Japanese researchers Ikemi and Nakagawa clearly demonstrated human susceptibility to both the positive and negative influences of a placebo.[11] In the study, thirteen boys with previously known reactions to the toxic leaves of lacquer trees were told they were going to be exposed to them.

During the study, the boys were blindfolded while one of their arms was brushed with the lacquer tree leaves and the other arm was brushed with leaves of a different species that were known to have no adverse effects. But the researchers told them they were doing the *opposite* of what they were really doing. The arm they said was brushed with the leaves of the lacquer tree was actually brushed with the safe leaves, and vice versa.

Only two of the boys experienced a reaction on the arm that had been rubbed with the lacquer leaves, yet all thirteen subjects had skin reactions to the harmless leaves they had been told were the harmful ones.

Fascinated by results like this—studies proving our minds have some type of power over our physical health—I pushed myself and focused my mind with every bit of inner strength

I had to believe that I was already healed. I also widened my research to include anything I could find about the mind, from neuroscience to quantum healing to metaphysics, and everything in between.

I read for hours a day and for days on end, searching for anything that talked about the potential power to heal. Eager to get my life back, I tried any suggested healing modality that I came across. Yet no matter what I did, I could not get my body to heal. At times when I was in deep states of meditation, my pain decreased while other times it wouldn't budge. I would make some progress but always experienced setbacks.

One year passed, then another and another. It became difficult to make myself believe each day that I was healed already because the pain was still ever-present.

IT BECAME CLEAR THERE WERE FACTORS OTHER THAN BELIEF

As I researched the "power of belief" more deeply, I began to see that I didn't have the full picture when it came to the success of the placebo; there were other factors to consider. For example, research has shown that the effectiveness of the placebo increases when there is a caring doctor–patient relationship.[12]

I was surprised to find a lesser-known type of placebo called the "open-label placebo," or "nonblind" placebo. This is a study on the placebo where both the doctor and the patient know that the treatment is a fake, yet researchers have still been able to document real physiological changes.

The first recorded study I could find on the open-label placebo took place in 1963 in the outpatient department of the Henry Phipps Psychiatric Clinic. The objective was to test the efficacy of a nonblind placebo on patients who were suffering from mental illness with signs of anxiety.

Due to the unorthodox nature of the study, it was limited to only fifteen patients. Each patient was asked to discontinue any antidepressants, tranquilizers, or sedatives to ensure that they would take only the placebo. Then they were scheduled for two appointments. The initial one was a regular new patient consultation in which the patient was evaluated by the doctor for about an hour. But at the end of the appointment, the doctor carefully followed a script that, in short, suggested to the patient that they should take the placebo because it may help give them some relief. The script also included telling the patient the placebo was merely a "sugar pill" that contained no medicine, yet it had helped others with their condition regardless.[13]

The patient was then given a bottle of placebo pills with the label from Johns Hopkins on it. Each was instructed to take one placebo capsule three times per day with meals for one week. Then they were to return for their follow-up appointment.

One week later, when the participants arrived for the follow-up appointment, fourteen out of the fifteen patients had taken the capsules. Surprisingly, *all fourteen* had shown improvement in at least one area. On average, the improvement was significant, with the average decrease in symptoms of 41 percent!

Also fascinating was that at the end of the study, the researchers asked each of the participants what they believed caused the results. Some stated they believed the improvements were not connected to the pill. Others fully believed they were taking a placebo; therefore the placebo must have helped. And six of the participants, despite the script, believed the placebo had real medicine in it. Interestingly, the study states, "There was no difference in improvement ratings between those eight patients who believed the pills contained placebo and the six patients who believed an active drug was involved."

The open-label placebo is a rapidly growing area of interest with a number of studies that demonstrate this incredible phenomenon. For example, a 2010 study on the open-label placebo was entitled, "Placebos Without Deception: A Randomized Controlled Trial in Irritable Bowel Syndrome."[14] In this, the researchers noted that those who were given the open-label placebo reported several improvements, including a reduction in the severity of IBS symptoms.

The more I learned about both the placebo and the open-label placebo, it became evident that the physical changes could not be solely due to belief. There had to be something else happening in the mind.

Furthermore, if belief really *was* the only factor needed for the mind to heal the body, shouldn't it have worked for me already? I had tried a vast number of treatments, prescription drugs, procedures, herbs, supplements, and other alternative remedies I believed would work. And while some things helped a bit, none of them had healed my body.

THE POWER OF THE MIND TO AFFECT THE BODY WITHOUT BELIEF

One area of research that was eye-opening for me had been conducted on people who suffered from dissociative identity disorder (DID), formerly known as multiple personality disorder (MPD). Studies showed that different alters (alternate personalities or identities) sharing the same physical body could have very different biomarkers and even different ailments. For example, as each personality assumed control of the shared body, it could have different temperatures, blood pressures, and heart rates. One personality may suffer from headaches, asthma, allergies, or pain, but an alternate personality may not suffer from any physical ailments at all.[15,16]

There is also a well-known case where a blind woman with multiple personalities had the ability to see in some of her alternate personalities (alters).[17,18]

The mere fact that incurable medical conditions could change between alters was remarkable. It hinted that it was *possible* to heal ailments considered "incurable" by conventional medical standards. The more I researched, the more I questioned what I thought I knew about health and our physical bodies.

One by one, I analyzed every medical anomaly I could find, including a phenomenon called "phantom pain," which is when a person missing a limb experiences intermittent physical pain in that area. Research shows that more than 80 percent of amputees can experience phantom pain.[19]

I also became fascinated with spontaneous healing, or spontaneous remission, which is when symptoms disappear, and a person can be listed as medically cured from their illnesses without any formal treatment.[20]

The Institute of Noetic Sciences published a book called *Spontaneous Remission: An Annotated Bibliography*, which became known as "the largest collection of medically documented cases of spontaneous remission in the world" with more than 3,500 references.[21]

I was perplexed. How was it possible for the body to heal from an incurable condition without any identifiable cause? It was clear that if I was going to figure out how to heal,

I needed a more logical understanding of how the mind and body's natural healing processes worked.

During my career in network operations, most of my days had been spent testing and troubleshooting communication networks. I knew from years of experience that when it came to complex issues, if I first simplified the issue down to its smallest building blocks, I could build on each piece of the puzzle until I found the solution.

I also knew that if I started with the most complex parts of the problem—the unknowns and anomalies—then I would likely stay stuck without answers, which is exactly what I had been doing.

While my research had been helpful up to this point because I could see evidence proving that our minds could affect our physical health, I felt it was time to change my approach. I decided to go back to doing things the way I knew worked best: simplifying everything until the answers became evident.

And just as I hoped, this approach soon revealed some extremely helpful information for me and many others.

3

SEEING THE LIGHT:
A NEW WAY TO LOOK
AT YOUR HEALTH

*The ability to simplify means to eliminate the unnecessary
so that the necessary may speak.*

—Hans Hoffman[1]

In order to simplify each data point and figure out what might
be missing, I took a step back from the bigger picture and began
analyzing the daily regimen I had created for myself. It included
a variety of healthy practices such as meditating for several
hours per day, listening to special healing music, trying different
diets, and taking handfuls of supplements. I had been following
this routine for several years, even adding in occasional fasting
and detoxing, yet my body wasn't healing.

My initial thought behind this approach was that either
I would experience a spontaneous remission, or that this daily
regimen would radically speed up the rate at which my body

repaired itself, going beyond its everyday restorative ability to heal my serious injuries.

As I analyzed my intentions, I realized that I needed to do more than just focus on speeding up my body's ability to heal. After all, my body's natural healing system appeared to be functioning well. For example, if I had a minor cut it would heal as expected. And even after getting nerve ablations, my nerves had grown back. These were just some of the signs that showed me that my body's natural healing system was generally working as it should. This led me to the conclusion that I would need to target the specific areas of my body that needed healing.

But the key question remained: *Why would some parts of my body heal but not others?*

YOUR BODY'S NATURAL ABILITY TO SELF-REPAIR

As I was analyzing the body's natural healing system, it became clear to me that our bodies are in a constant state of repairing, renewing, and replacing cells. For example, research estimates that we shed about 40,000 skin cells every minute and renew our outermost layer of skin approximately every thirty days.[2] Inside the body, approximately 330 billion cells die every day, which are then replaced by new ones.[3] Even our bones are steadily renewing themselves through a process called bone remodeling. It's estimated that the skeleton almost completely regenerates, or remodels itself, approximately every ten years.[4,5]

Under certain circumstances, the body even seems to be able to repair DNA damage fairly quickly. For example, research has concluded that when a person engages in intense exercise, it creates DNA damage. Yet this damage is typically repaired within twenty-four to seventy-two hours.[6]

Leaving no stone unturned, I continued to research the renewal rates of the physical body in hopes of discovering a clue on how I might be able to use this information to heal myself. Eventually, I came across an article in *Time* magazine from 1954 called "Science: The Fleeting Flesh." In it, Dr. Paul C. Aebersold from Oak Ridge National Laboratory shared his research, revealing that approximately 98 percent of the atoms in the human body are renewed each year.[7] This was also published in the *Annual Report* of the Smithsonian Institution.

As I read Aebersold's research and analyzed the rate of renewal of the body, I began to reflect on how long I'd been injured, which was sobering for several reasons. I could see just how much I'd been living life in my head to the point I had lost touch with time. I was obsessed with healing. It was the only thing that mattered. I spent every waking moment I could working on healing in one way or another: researching, meditating, writing affirmations, doing as much as I could when I could. I was afraid to stop. Even in the presence of others, the voice inside my head was the loudest in the room. I was caught up in a constant stream of thoughts, telling myself I was already healed.

Sleepless nights transitioned to daybreak as I could see the first morning light come through the windows. Another morning always came and went, leaving me without answers. I began to calculate the years that had passed. It had been almost five years since my injury; it felt like an eternity. I didn't recognize my life and couldn't help but feel discouraged. I was doing literally everything I could think of. If my body was replacing 98 percent of the atoms each year, I couldn't understand why it wasn't healing itself. It was a thought that was stuck in my head every day, which only led to more questions.

If my body regularly renews and repairs itself, then why, after all these years, would my body not heal itself? How was it possible for a person to have an illness or injury continue for ten, twenty, or even fifty years?

Questioning my health from all angles, I wondered if certain parts of my body were not repairing or renewing. Or, if by chance, my body was in a cycle and recreating illness? And if so, why? It was an odd thought. I wondered if my brain had a blueprint for my body, and if illness was somehow included in that blueprint—in which case, my body's renewal system continued to recreate the problem.

Aebersold's article spurred my journey toward studying atoms and molecules and, following that, toward a deep exploration of the energy of the body.

LIGHT ENERGY AND CELL PROLIFERATION

The concept of energy in the body has been well-documented for thousands of years in Chinese medicine as well as through several religious and spiritual teachings. While some people believe that energy is simply a spiritual or metaphysical belief, it turns out that science has also documented that the cells of all living organisms really do emit a type of light energy.[8,9]

Throughout the years, this light energy has been called by several different names. When it was first scientifically discovered in the 1920s by biologist and medical scientist Alexander Gurwitsch, he named it "mitogenetic radiation." However, as additional discoveries were made, the name also evolved and today this light energy is now most commonly referred to as biophotons or Ultra-Weak Photon Emission (UPE). For simplicity, I'll generally refer to it as biophotons, or simply as "light energy."

Gurwitsch received an outpouring of recognition for discovering this incredible light energy and was even nominated for a Nobel Prize eleven times.[10] In 1941, he was awarded the USSR State Prize[11] (similar to the Nobel Prize for the Soviet Union) because this light energy led to a less-expensive method to detect and diagnose cancer.[12,13]

I was drawn to Gurwitsch's research for one primary reason: he'd been able to demonstrate this light energy could increase *cell proliferation*, which is the growth and division of cells to create more cells.[14,15] (An easy way to picture cell proliferation would be to imagine a golf ball as the cell, growing and dividing into two full-size golf balls, which then grow and divide into four, then eight, and so on.) The fact that this light energy could influence cell proliferation drew my attention for several reasons:

- Healthy cell proliferation is needed for growth, healing, and immune system regulation in the human body[16–19]
- Slow cell growth and division can result in a slower, decreased ability to heal[20]
- Research has shown that decreased, abnormal, or excessive cell proliferation can be a key factor in many diseases.[21–23]

It may sound odd that this light energy can help the growth and division of cells inside our bodies, but an easy way to illustrate the power of light is to imagine a plant under grow lights. With the right amount of light, the plant will grow.

To demonstrate the impact of this light energy in his experiments, Gurwitsch used a tube to funnel this light energy from one onion root (the *emitter* of energy) through a tube onto a second onion root (the *receiver* of the energy). Think of it like a thin pipe (or a very weak light laser) placed between two onions. The results showed that the location on the onion root that *directly received* this light energy had an increased number of cells growing and dividing. The fact that this light energy influenced cell proliferation was profound.

I began to wonder, *Why don't more people know that our bodies emit light energy? Why is this not common knowledge?*

After more research, it appeared that the answer might be, in part, because a significant amount of research on the human body has been conducted using cadavers. And while the information gleaned from cadavers has been crucial to the medical field, cadavers obviously don't emit any light energy (only living cells do).[24,25] Furthermore, because this light energy is weak and invisible, it's hard to test. In most cases, to accurately measure this light energy from the body, researchers must be in a pitch-black room with special equipment. Given these factors, the majority of medical studies have been completed without ever taking into consideration that this light is emitted throughout our bodies.

In fact, testing has historically been part of the problem with this light energy. After Gurwitsch completed his experiments, the results generated a lot of excitement among other medical scientists and researchers; however, they initially failed to duplicate his results so his discovery was largely forgotten until many years later.

DISCOVERING BIOPHOTONS

As technology advanced and testing evolved, this light energy was confirmed by German biophysicist Fritz-Albert Popp in the 1970s. He was able to validate and further build on Gurwitsch's discoveries. Popp found an even wider spectrum of light energy, as well as evidence that this light energy may also play a role in regulating all the life processes that occur in a biological organism. Instead of using the name *mitogenetic radiation*, Popp coined the term "biophotons."[26–28]

The easiest way to think about a biophoton is to first consider a regular photon, which is a light particle emitted by a nonliving source. (For simplicity, it might be useful to picture a tiny particle of light energy emitted by a light bulb.) In contrast, a biophoton is a particle of light emitted by a living biological source, such as a plant, animal, or human. Thus, the primary difference is the *source* of the light particle.

Since Popp's discovery, this light energy has been studied in universities around in the world, and there have been a range of new discoveries (including new research after my 2010 recovery),[29–34] which I will share in the upcoming pages.

While there is still so much unknown about light energy (biophotons), the foundational discoveries that most researchers agree on are that it:

- Plays an important role in supporting the basic functions of all cells[35,36]
- Supports communication between cells[37–43]
- Can influence cell growth and division[44–48]
- Participates in neural signal transmission and processing.[49–52]

It was interesting to think about this light energy communicating information throughout our bodies. After all, having worked in telecommunications, I was well aware that light energy is used in communication around the world through fiber-optic cables. For example, the internet, television, and cell phones often use light in fiber optics to communicate, which is part of the reason that a person can receive an email, text message, or other media message instantly—pretty much at the speed of light!

While researchers have provided clear evidence that cells use light energy to communicate, it seems that the outcome may not always be a positive one. Furthermore, studies also reveal that there is a correlation between certain illnesses and light energy.

DIFFERENT ENERGY PATTERNS CORRELATE WITH DIFFERENT ILLNESSES

Studies have found that different illnesses emit different light energy. In a 2004 study, researchers were exploring the use of biophotons as a novel technique for cancer imaging and found that "the intensity of biophoton emission reflects the viability of the tumor tissue."[53]

Additionally, in a 2018 study, researchers documented the specific biophoton markers of malignant cells. Their results revealed that the biophoton emissions from cancerous cells had notably different patterns and wavelengths versus noncancerous cells.[54,55]

These variations are seen not only in cancerous cells though. In a groundbreaking 2016 study, researchers studied biophoton emissions from patients with type 2 diabetes and sought to establish evidence that biophotons could be used as a noninvasive diagnostic tool.[56] In their study, they compared biophoton emissions from sixty healthy patients to biophoton emissions of fifty patients with type 2 diabetes and found that there was a significant difference between the two groups.

The researchers noted that the average biophoton intensity of the navel area was significantly higher in the diabetic group than in the healthy group.[57] However, the intensity of biophoton emission was higher in the forehead and throat areas for the group of healthy individuals than it was for the diabetic group.

What does all this mean? When a person has an illness, the light energy in their body changes. Not only can the *intensity* of biophoton emission from the cells change but there can also be a difference in the location of the body from which it is being emitted.

Thanks to studies such as this one, researchers are working toward collecting enough data to integrate light energy into our medical system as an alternative type of noninvasive early detection diagnostic tool. While these studies are incredible and exciting, more progress remains to be made in the area of biophoton research in general. Though researchers have been able to identify patterns of biophoton emission, to date, there is still no way to fully "decrypt" this light energy.[58]

A simple way to think about identifying patterns and interpreting this light energy is to first recall that the body can use this light energy to communicate. As a metaphor, you could imagine that all of the cells of the body are sending emails to each other written in a foreign language. At this time, researchers cannot interpret this language; therefore they cannot read the information being sent. However, by analyzing multiple emails and noting the patterns—such as repeated letters, numbers, or symbols, or that some emails are similar to one another while others are distinctly different—researchers could compare the emails and identify patterns associated with certain illnesses. Continuing with this analogy, they may look for differences in the patterns and notice higher intensity emails from cancer cells. And with type 2 diabetes, they may find a higher rate of emails being sent in one area of the body, which is distinctly different from someone who is healthy or without type 2 diabetes.

POSITIVE AND NEGATIVE EFFECTS OF LIGHT ENERGY

In my situation, instead of thinking about biophotons in terms of *diagnostics*, since I already had a diagnosis, I was asking myself different questions: *What if light energy was the key to activating the body's self-healing mechanism? What if light energy was also a hidden factor in the creation of illness?*

To be clear, this is not to say that light energy is bad. After all, research suggested that this light energy plays a role in supporting several functions of our cells. However, the more I analyzed the data, the more it appeared as though light energy may have the potential to exert either a positive *or* negative influence on the cells.

A 2009 study by Sergey Mayburov at the Lebedev Institute of Physics showed just that. It involved a series of experiments analyzing the communication and the effects of light energy on fish eggs and frog eggs. The results showed that when light energy was emitted from one type of egg and transmitted onto other eggs, it could have a physical influence on the cells and change the growth rates. In some cases, this light energy could increase cell growth and division. In other cases, he noted that the light energy led to "serious deformation of development" and could even stop development completely.[59]

Looking at the collective data, research suggests that light energy, in general, can:

- Exert positive or negative effects on cell growth and division
- Communicate vital information throughout the body, including reestablishing homeostasis, which is important for healing[60,61] (simply stated, homeostasis is the body's ability to maintain a stable balance needed for survival)
- Have a dramatic influence on biochemical reactivity[62-64]
- Transmit along neural fibers and take part in neural signal transmission and processing.[65-67]

The more I explored this light energy, the more it felt like I was on the verge of a major breakthrough. All the evidence pointed to biophotons as holding an important key to healing, as well as possibly being a hidden culprit behind illness.

4

YOUR MIND'S ABILITY
TO INFLUENCE
LIGHT ENERGY

We speak about feeling, because knowledge alone
cannot provide an understanding of energy.

—Koot Hoomi[1]

As I pored over research, reading everything I could about light energy, I kept my mind open for any clues about how I could use this information to heal myself. Eventually, I came across studies that revealed an astonishing breakthrough: Our own thoughts and emotions have the ability to influence light energy.

The first study I found revealing that brain activity could influence biophotons was completed on laboratory rats back in 1995. In that study, researchers discovered a correlation between the intensity of biophoton emission and changes in neural activity.[2,3]

It seemed to me that if it were possible for a rat's brain to influence light energy (biophotons), then surely it must be possible for a human brain to do the same. I searched for any new or obscure studies I could find on the topic, which ultimately revealed it was indeed possible![4-6]

Between the years of 2005 and 2008, several groundbreaking studies were conducted on people who were using various forms of meditation and relaxation techniques. In each of these studies, researchers measured biophoton emission from the particpiants and discovered that these types of activities could decrease biophoton emission.[7-10] It was noted that biophoton emission decreased not only in the head, but also throughout other locations of the body as well.

Over the years, research continued to corroborate that our minds can influence biophoton emission not only through relaxation and meditation but in a variety of different and specific ways. For instance, in a 2011 study, researchers asked participants to visualize white light. As they did, biophoton emission increased from the right side of the participant's head but not the left. The authors noted that mundane or ordinary thinking didn't seem to have a major influence, producing no change in biophoton emission on either side of the head.[11]

In another study in 2021, researchers examined the effects of anger on biophoton emission. Their research revealed that when volunteers were experiencing strong feelings of anger, the intensity of biophoton emission from the volunteer's torso was notably higher compared to when the volunteers were in a relaxed state.[12]

Since the research showed that relaxation led to decreased biophoton emission, and that increased brain activity and emotions were linked to increased biophoton emission, I began looking at the connection between light energy and emotions in an effort to better understand the correlation.

Note: At some point, you may begin to wonder if there is a difference between an *emotion* and a *feeling*. The technical answer is yes. However, defining the difference could add an additional layer of complexity that is not needed. For this reason, I will be using the terms interchangeably throughout this book. (If you would like more information on the difference between emotions and feelings, you can find a link on the website for this book at brandygillmore.com/bookbonuses).

CONNECTING THE DOTS BETWEEN BIOPHOTONS AND EMOTIONS

As I began researching thoughts and emotions, I didn't just search for general information on psychological stress. Instead, I approached my research in a very specific way because, despite the wealth of data proving that stress could impact our health, I could objectively see that something was missing.

I pondered the fact that many people living seemingly low-stress lives with very positive attitudes can nonetheless struggle with major and even terminal health issues. On the flip side, there are also people with high levels of stress suffering from extreme trauma who have no physical health issues at all. For example, I could observe the fact that some police officers who had been diagnosed with PTSD had major health issues, yet many others who suffered from PTSD had none. Based on this, it seemed to me that while the level of stress may be a factor, clearly it was not the *sole* factor causing pain or illness.

However, since research has revealed that our thoughts and emotions can influence light energy, and that light energy can influence cell growth and division, I connected the dots and began to look for the direct line of evidence that connected our thoughts and emotions to cell growth and division (proliferation). I figured that if these were indeed connected, then surely there must be proven research revealing this connection. It was easy to see that there was!

Studies proved increased stress can:

- Lower immune proliferation responses[13,14]
- Increase cancer proliferation and progression[15,16]
- Decrease general levels of cell growth and division, which can be associated with both accelerated aging and slower healing rates[17–19]
- Affect post-surgical results. People who have surgery while experiencing feelings of fear or distress can experience slower healing, poorer outcomes, longer recovery times, greater chances of postoperative complications, and higher rates of re-hospitalization than people in a positive state of mind.[20,21]

As I read through one study after another, it was easy to see the direct link between stress (negative emotions) and proliferation (cell growth and division). And because research showed that biophotons could either positively or negatively influence cell growth and division, I intentionally sought out studies that also included the positive effects of emotions, too.

Research revealed that optimism can speed up healing and postsurgical recovery times and even help protect against illness and death.[22] A fifteen-year study completed in 2007 showed that "emotional vitality" (defined as "a sense of energy, positive well-being, and effective emotion regulation") may even protect against the risk of coronary heart disease.[23] Furthermore, a

2019 study researching the connection between optimism and longevity found that people who were classified as "more optimistic" can live up to 15 percent longer than those who were classified as the "least optimistic."[24,25]

While I had known previously that emotions could influence our health, I hadn't fully realized the significant impact they could have on light energy. Nor had I fully grasped that our invisible emotions could affect cell growth and division.

This was eye-opening as to the level of influence that emotions can have on our healing, illness, and even longevity!

ARE BIOPHOTONS THE MISSING (INVISIBLE) PIECE OF THE HEALING PUZZLE?

Thinking back over every one of the medical mysteries I'd been researching, it seemed as though each one could theoretically make sense if I factored the power of emotions and biophotons into the equation.

Analyzing the Placebo Effect Through a New Lens: The Biophoton-Placebo Theory

One of the aspects I'd found puzzling about a placebo was how it was possible for it to have a *specific* effect on the physical body. As we discussed previously on p21, if a person were told that a placebo could improve their symptoms of Parkinson's disease, then it could. If instead they were told the placebo would reduce their high blood pressure, then it actually could reduce their blood pressure significantly.[26] In the case of the nocebo, if a patient were told there would be specific negative side effects, the person could experience those exact side effects.

I'd been stumped about how it was possible for the specific information that a person was told to be communicated to the cells of the body. However, after studying biophotons, it appeared that they could hold the key. Research has revealed that biophotons can communicate information throughout the body. This includes vital information about the body's health.

Additionally, when it comes to the effects of the placebo, it is well-documented that emotions can play a significant role. For example:

- Studies from as far back as 1969 suggest that if a person expects a positive outcome from taking the placebo, this expectation can reduce their negative stressful emotions, which can create physiological changes.[27]
- A caring doctor–patient relationship can have a significant impact on the outcome of the placebo.[28]
- Feelings of positive expectation from the placebo can trigger the release of positive biochemicals in the brain.[29]

Since research has shown that biophotons have the ability to communicate information to cells and also play an important role in biochemical changes, it made logical sense that the combination of emotions and biophotons could indeed be the hidden culprits behind the placebo effect.[30,31]

A New Perspective on MPD/DID: Biophoton-Multiple Personality Theory

When I first came across research revealing that a person with multiple personalities could have specific illnesses in their host personality (their main personality), but not have any health issues (or entirely different health issues) in their alternate personalities, it was perplexing as to how that could be possible. However, it seemed that this phenomenon could be explained because different alters can have radically different emotional states. In fact, research has shown that EEG brain scans from different alters (personalities) can have significant differences.[32]

This could, in turn, result in radical changes in a person's brain chemistry and biophoton emission.

A New Hypothesis on Spontaneous Healing
In the case of spontaneous remission (spontaneous healing), it seemed that if a person had a strong emotional change, or "change of heart," this this could create a genuine shift in their thoughts and emotions that could also cause a shift in their biophoton emission and brain chemistry. This would be akin to a person who had MPD/DID switching to an alter with no health issues (as discussed on p26), but then never returning to the personality that suffered from health issues.

The Connection Between Biophotons (Light Energy) and Free Radicals
It's agreed upon by most medical researchers that there's a link between illness and free radicals. If you're not familiar with free radicals, they are atoms with an unpaired (uneven) number of electrons. An easy way to think about free radicals is to picture a car with an uneven number of tires (imagine the car has two or three tires instead of four tires). As a result, it's unstable and driving out of control, attempting to steal a tire from another car, and in the process, damaging other cars. Similarly, free radicals try to steal an electron from cells in the body and, in doing so, they can create damage inside the body.

While many people attribute free radicals (also called oxidative stress) to toxins such as pollution, chemicals, and pesticides, research has also shown that psychological stress can be a factor in their creation.[33] Further, there's a clear connection between stress, free radicals, and biophotons. One study specifically states, "This association between stress, ROS generation [free radicals], and biophoton emission is well-documented, and numerous researchers, including us, consider that the stress levels of living organisms can be inferred in real time by measuring biophoton emission."[34-37]

Reviewing each of the medical mysteries that had previously stumped me, I came to a realization: if I looked at them with emotions and biophotons as part of the equation, each of them could make logical sense!

THE CHALLENGES WITH INTEGRATING LIGHT ENERGY

The more I viewed everything through this lens, the more I saw the synergistic connection between emotions, biophotons, and health, which was exciting. If you're like me, having gained this knowledge, you may wonder, *Why haven't biophotons been integrated into our medical system?*

I could see a few possible reasons for this: the first and most obvious goes back to the awareness that most people don't know that biophotons exist. Secondly, most medical studies never consider this light energy, so it's essentially ignored as a variable. There's also the fact that some research is still conducted using cadavers, which obviously don't emit any light energy. Additionally, light energy can be laborious to test. But even when it's tested, we still can't see the full picture because according to 2011 research: "the highest intensity of biophotons cannot be measured because it is absorbed during cellular processes."[38,39] So even though this light energy was medically discovered more than a hundred years ago, and we know that it has the ability to communicate important information and influence the growth and division of cells, currently there is no way to interpret it or fully test it. (Note: Although it was not possible to test this mind-body-biophoton hypothesis due to the inability to fully test light energy, I discovered an alternative method to visually demonstrate the healing potential of the mind-body connection using medical thermal imaging which I will share with you in the upcoming pages.)

Despite the challenges with testing, there is some progress toward integrating light energy/biophotons into our medical system. Since researchers have been able to document the connection between biophotons and illness, they are working to identify the specific patterns that are associated with different illnesses. Their goal is to create a database for an early detection diagnostic tool.[40]

There are other ways we can observe efforts to try to use the power of light energy for healing as well. In fact, several top hospitals around the world have begun offering alternative services for energy healing by having one person use their hands to send energy to another.[41-44] Lasers are also being used as an alternative therapy for a variety of common issues, such as wound healing, pain and inflammation reduction, and to stimulate cell proliferation. Researchers suggest that this type of external light therapy, or photobiomodulation, engages the body's "biophoton code."[45] However, there is some mixed research on laser therapy. Because this light energy can increase cell proliferation, researchers also suggest that if a person has cancer, under certain conditions, it could potentially increase the proliferation of cancer cells.[46,47]

For me personally, knowing that even light energy from fish eggs could produce positive or negative effects on other eggs (as discussed on p38), and that we're still unable to fully interpret/decode the body's own self-produced light energy, I was not keen on the idea of receiving external treatments. And I didn't want to wait another hundred years, or however long it took until someone could fully test and decrypt it, if ever. On top of that, I was not in need of another diagnosis. I had plenty. I just wanted to heal as quickly as possible. Since research had revealed that our own minds have the ability to influence this incredible light energy, I continued down the rabbit hole to figure out how I could use this information and the power of my own mind to heal myself.

5

A DEEPER LEVEL
OF THE MIND

Many people think that the progress of the human race is based
on experiences of an empirical, critical nature, but I say that true
knowledge is to be had only through a philosophy of deduction.

—Albert Einstein[1]

The more I grasped the magnitude that our thoughts and emotions have the ability to influence biophoton emission and even affect cell proliferation, the more I began to see emotions in a radically new way. They weren't simply emotions; they were far more powerful than I had initially given them credit for.

I started to wonder how many illnesses could be linked in one way or another to psychological stress (negative emotions). One by one, I began researching every illness I could find from A to Z. I began with *abdominal aortic aneurysm, acne, acute cholecystitis, acute lymphoblastic leukemia,* and so on throughout the entire alphabet. I found scientific research on virtually every illness revealing that psychological stress could, in some way, directly or indirectly, affect or exacerbate the illness. Even those I wouldn't have initially considered to be influenced by stress, such as bone loss, hearing loss, and loss of eyesight, have been linked to stress.[2,3]

But when it came to the idea of healing with emotions, I thought back to the awareness that happy people could also suffer from health issues. Clearly there had to be other factors to consider.

A SIMPLE OBSERVATION OF THE IMPACT OF EMOTIONS

Using my approach of starting with the simplest known facts, I began to examine the most basic ways that emotions could produce tangible effects in the physical body. I thought of how feeling embarrassed can cause visible blushing or feelings of nervousness can result in a "nervous stomach" or "butterflies," which can result in experiencing digestive issues. Or, on a positive note, how sexual emotions can result in physical arousal. When I stopped and thought about it, it was fascinating that even our momentary feelings can produce tangible effects in the physical body.

As I analyzed these examples, it seemed evident that short-term changes in our emotions or feelings could cause short-term changes in our bodies. Therefore it seemed logical that if a long-term health issue was indeed linked to emotions, then it would need to be linked to long-term emotions or emotional patterns (feelings that were experienced frequently).

I questioned, *Was it possible that I had long-term negative emotional patterns in my subconscious mind that were affecting my physical body or keeping me from healing? Or did I harbor negative emotions after my injury that kept me from healing?*

Initially, I felt that I didn't have negative emotions buried in my subconscious mind since I was generally an optimistic person. And it didn't seem as if my emotions could be relevant to my injury because I'd had a physical accident (fall). However, recalling the research showing that negative emotions could prevent a person from healing after surgery, I began to rethink everything. From that perspective, it didn't really matter *how* my injury occurred. What mattered was the time after the injury and the fact that I didn't heal. And when it came to the subconscious mind, I had to admit that it would be impossible for me to say with certainty that I didn't harbor any hidden emotions that were affecting me. After all, as the word indicates, information in the subconscious mind is "below consciousness."

By this point, I had already been working with my subconscious mind for several years, visualizing and listening to a variety of recordings meant to help change my brain waves and reprogram my subconscious mind for healing. While these recordings and daily meditations had helped to calm my nervous system, they hadn't healed my body. However, since all evidence seemed to be pointing toward one's mindset and emotions, I let go of any resistance I had and, with an open mind, began delving deeper into understanding the subconscious mind.

THE HIDDEN POWER OF SUBCONSCIOUS EMOTIONS

An easy way to think about the subconscious mind is like the hard drive (storage) in a computer. Even though we can't see into our subconscious mind, it stores all our files and programs—all the skills, habits, and memories of things we have ever experienced, including emotions and emotional patterns. It also stores our automatic habits, such as tying our shoes or brushing our teeth, as well as the memories to help us build and retain daily skills, such as driving.

It may seem odd that we have subconscious emotions and habits that occur without conscious thought, but a large part of how we function in life is unconscious. If you think about many of the physical processes that are needed to maintain life, they, too, occur automatically without conscious thought, such as breathing, digesting food, and the beating of our hearts. The same is true when it comes to our mental processes. Many of our emotions and motivations occur subconsciously, which, unbeknownst to us, can control our behavior even though it may not feel that way.[4,5]

On one hand, it's exciting that we have this "programmable" hard drive. In theory, if a person's subconscious mind contained nothing but happy and loving memories, habits, goals, motivations, and emotions, then that person would be programmed for a happy, loving, harmonious, and successful life. On the other hand, if negative information was stored in the subconscious mind, it could have the opposite effect by holding on to hurt and wounding that could negatively influence a person's mindset. In short, the information in a person's subconscious mind shapes their daily thoughts, actions, and behaviors without them ever consciously realizing it.

Throughout history, unconscious/automatic behaviors have been referred to by a variety of terms. In the thirteenth century, when philosopher and theologian Saint Thomas Aquinas wrote about subconscious actions, he used the term "involuntary actions" because this emotional and/or physical behavior was exactly that: automatic based on our subconscious programming.[6,7]

While subconscious behaviors have been written about throughout history, the theory that memories, emotions, and motivations are stored in the subconscious mind was first made popular by Austrian neurologist Sigmund Freud, who some consider to be the "father of modern psychology."[8] While Freud didn't invent psychology, he coined the term "psychoanalysis" in 1896 and established it as an important method of therapy. (Technically, the subconscious activities of the mind could be further segmented into different levels by labeling them as preconscious, unconscious, or even superconscious. But for the sake of simplicity throughout this book, I will use the term *subconscious* to refer to anything in the mind that is below our conscious awareness.)

Freud's understanding of how to work with the subconscious mind provided a breakthrough for treating patients who were suffering from various forms of mental illness. He realized that many of their problems stemmed from deep within their subconscious mind and were therefore not consciously available to the patient. His treatment focused on being able to gain access to the information stored in this deeper part of the mind, which is why psychoanalysis can also be referred to as "depth psychology." Through his work, he showed that resolving a problem (or memory) rooted deep in the patient's subconscious mind was important for the mental health of the patient.

Our subconscious minds govern our habits, emotions, and automatic behaviors that shape every aspect of our lives. Therefore, the more a person can access the information in their subconscious mind and transform their underlying emotions, motivations, habits, and behaviors, the more they can change themselves and enhance their levels of overall happiness and success in life.[9,10]

I contemplated what would happen if I could access my own subconscious emotions and change them. Could this, in turn, allow my body to heal itself? And if so, which emotion(s) would I need to change?

That proved to be the key question.

THE "EMOTIONAL BRAIN INJURY"

As I pondered which subconscious emotion(s) could be affecting me, I recalled the simple awareness that each emotion can impact the physical body in a different way. Thinking back to the previous example, if a person experiences intense emotions of embarrassment, this could result in a blushing face. In contrast, if a person experiences feelings of anxiety, there is an entirely different physical response: a racing heart and shortness of breath (known as a panic/anxiety attack). These physical responses are not random occurrences. It was clear that each emotion could elicit a very different physical response.

While this was obvious, it was also an important detail. For healing, this meant it would be imperative for me to analyze individual emotions instead of using general terms like *stress*, since each individual emotion could have its own distinct and specific effect on the physical body.

I contemplated how it could be possible for different emotions to affect different parts or functions of the body. This led me to think about the mind-body connection in the case of a brain injury or even a stroke. It's well-documented that if a person suffers from either a brain injury or a stroke, this can also affect their physical body. For example, if a person has a "right hemisphere stroke" (a stroke on the right side of the brain), it can affect the left side of a person's body. Conversely, a "left hemisphere stroke" can affect the right side of their body as well as a person's speech, language, and vision. This shows that the location of the brain injury matters.

Based on this understanding, I questioned: *Could it be possible that a negative emotion acts in a similar manner to an "emotional injury" to the brain, so to speak? What if the emotion generates negative activity in certain parts of the brain, which, in turn, negatively impacts the part of the body that is connected to that part of the brain?*

In this case, I use the term "emotional brain injury" as a metaphor to illustrate the idea that we can have emotional activity in the brain that, in turn, affects our physical body. However, technically speaking, studies have revealed that traumatic emotional events (such as child abuse and PTSD from a car accident) can change our brain structure.[11–13] The fact that our own emotions possess the power to change the physical structure of our brains was eye-opening.

THE MIND-BODY EMOTIONAL CONNECTION

I continued to think about the analogy of the "emotional injury" to the brain which led me to study the connection between the brain and body. This led me back to the well-known mind-body map (more formally known as the cortical homunculus; see illustration on p58) created in 1937 by neurosurgeon Wilder Penfield and Professor of Neurosurgery Edwin Boldrey. For simplicity, I'll refer to it as the "brain-body map."

This map is a neurological illustration that reveals how each part of the body is connected to a different location in the brain for sensory information and movement.[14] (Note: I share this illustration not because you need to know all of the specific locations in the brain, but to provide you with a visual image showing that each part of the body is connected to a different location in the brain.)

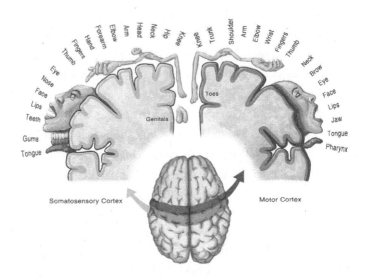

Illustration of the cortical homunculus originally created by Penfield and Boldrey: a visual representation that illustrates how different parts of the body are connected to different locations in the brain.[15]

As you look at this brain-body map, it's also interesting to note that research has revealed that emotions generate activity in the somatosensory cortex (which is on the left side of the image) and has even suggested that the somatosensory cortex is involved in every stage of emotional processing.[16] Given that each part of the physical body is connected to the somatosensory cortex, this was profound.

The more I thought about the mind-body connection and the cortical homunculus, the more I started to see how it might be possible to heal myself. But it wasn't just the brain-body map itself that was so insightful; it was also the *process* the researchers used to create the map.

To create the map, researchers stimulated different locations in their patients' brains and then documented which part of the physical body was affected by the brain stimulation. Following this protocol, they were able to create the first brain-body map.

What is also important to note is that patients didn't merely report a vague sensation in their body; they could experience a variety of specific physical reactions. For example, Penfield documented that when he probed an area of the brain called the insular cortex, patients could feel nauseated, gassy, bloated, or even ready to vomit.[17]

Based on this awareness, it again made me wonder if emotions could do the same thing and, in short, *act in a similar way to electrical stimulation, whereby they could fire in the brain and in turn impact the corresponding part of the physical body.*

As I continued to analyze the mind-body connection from this perspective, I came across research that could support it. For example, there was a case study of a thirty-year-old man who suffered from extreme fear, tightness in his throat, seizures, and projectile vomiting. When researchers monitored his brain, they saw spikes in a specific location of his brain: the insular cortex. At the direction of his doctors, the patient then underwent a temporal lobectomy, which included removing that specific portion of his brain. After doing so, both the seizures and vomiting completely stopped.[18]

While I am definitely not a proponent of practices such as these, the evidence from this case study was profound. The researchers noted that the insular cortex appeared to be a specific trigger area for vomiting. This was consistent with Penfield's research. Furthermore, the researchers also documented that the patient struggled with an intense emotion: *fear.*

Of course, this is not the only link between fear and vomiting. It's well-documented that people who suffer from extreme panic attacks can feel queasy, experience nausea, or sometimes even vomit. Common examples may include people who experience fear of public speaking or fear of flying in an airplane. As a result, they may feel nauseous, which could potentially result in vomiting.

As I continued to analyze emotions and health from this perspective, I could see with even more clarity as to how it was possible for inexplicable anomalies to make *logical* sense.

Referring back to MPD/DID, the fact that a person could suffer from headaches in one personality (alter), and asthma or chronic pain in another personality (alter), but have no symptoms or health issues in another alter could make logical sense.[19] After all, if different emotions were stimulating different parts of the brain, which, in turn, were affecting different parts of the physical body, then as a person with MPD/DID changed alters, it would make logical sense that it could affect different parts of the body depending upon which emotions a person was feeling. No matter how I looked at it, everything seemed to be pointing me in one direction: our thoughts and emotions hold the key.

A QUICK PIVOT BACK TO LIGHT ENERGY

In thinking about the brain-body map, the fact that Penfield and Boldrey used electrical stimulation, which travelled from the brain down neural fibers to affect the corresponding part of the body, intrigued me. Theoretically, if electrical stimulation can travel from the brain to the body this way, then biophotons (light energy) should be able to do the same. After all, research has shown that biophotons can transmit along neural fibers, too.[20]

What is also very interesting is that if this light energy did travel to a specific location in the body (similar to Penfield and Boldrey's research), then theoretically it would be much stronger than regular energy because it would be "funneled."

An easy way to think about "funneled" light energy is to imagine the sun, a magnifying glass, and a piece of paper. In ordinary daylight, the sun's energy would not ignite the piece of paper. But if a person were to hold a magnifying glass with the sun's rays focused on a specific spot on the paper, it could start a fire. This occurs because a magnifying glass collects the photons and "funnels" them to a single point. We can see this is true with biophotons as well. If you recall the experiment with the onions, light energy was funneled through a tube from one onion onto another. This resulted in cell proliferation on the specific part of the onion that was receiving the light energy. Similarly, if light energy (biophotons) was traveling from the brain to the body, this could "funnel" light energy all to one location (similar to the electrical stimulation that was used to create the brain-body map).

The more I thought about it, the more I could see that there were several ways in which this light energy could affect the human body. While I yearned to be able to fully test biophotons, I could also see that I didn't really need to. After all, there was a *substantial* body of evidence which proved that our own thoughts and emotions could impact our health. With this in mind, I continued to analyze my "emotional brain injury" metaphor and the brain-body map. It seemed that there must be a "brain-emotion-body" connection.

EMOTIONS GENERATING ACTIVITY THROUGHOUT THE BRAIN

In the time that has lapsed since my 2010 recovery, there have been several cutting-edge studies that have used functional magnetic resonance imaging (fMRI) scans to document the activity that emotions generate in the brain.

One groundbreaking study conducted by researchers at Carnegie Mellon University has revealed that different emotions do indeed generate activity in different parts of the brain. And the same emotions generate activity in the same parts of the brain.[21]

In this study, participants were asked to go through a series of different emotions repeatedly, in random order, while scientists used functional magnetic resonance imaging (fMRI) and machine learning to analyze their brain activity. Results showed that if two people were experiencing the same emotion (e.g., both people experiencing fear) their brain scans were similar to one another. However, if two people were experiencing different emotions, such as one feeling happy and the other sad, their brain scans were distinctly different from one another.

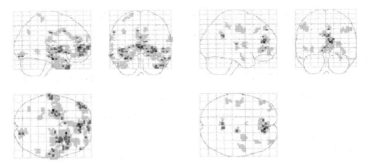

Brain images taken by researchers at Carnegie Mellon University depict that emotions can generate neural activity throughout a number of brain regions.[22]

It is also interesting to note—based on the brain scans in this study—that emotions generate activity throughout the brain, not in just one location. One of the researchers, Vladimir Cherkassky, stated, "This suggests that emotion signatures aren't limited to specific brain regions, such as the amygdala, but produce characteristic patterns throughout a number of brain regions."[23] (See the brain scan images opposite.)

Based on this research, we can see how it would be possible for the same emotion to physically affect two people in the same way. Recalling the stroke discussion (and "emotional brain injury" metaphor), if two people have a right brain stroke, they could be physically affected in a similar way because the same part of the brain is affected (the right hemisphere).

Now if we look at emotions in the same way, two people could have the same response to an emotion for the same reason: because the same part of the brain is affected. And, since a different emotion would generate activity in a different area of the brain, we can see how a different emotion could produce a different physical effect.

It was interesting to note that the researchers from this study also concluded that the neural signatures of positive emotions were distinctly different from the neural signatures that were associated with negative emotions.

Of course, as I read their research it made me wonder if this is the reason that positive emotions have a significantly different effect on the physical body than negative emotions.

THE POWER OF SPECIFIC EMOTIONS

Making a point to return to the simplest known facts, I began looking at how individual emotions can create obvious specific and consistent physical effects. I considered the example of a person having the feeling of being embarrassed; this emotion consistently links to a blushing face. It does not, however, link to a panic attack unless the person experiences feelings of panic. As I thought about individual emotions, it was clear that each emotion affected the body in its own way. This was not only true for visible physical reactions, such as embarrassment or anxiety, but also for things we can't see, like biochemical reactions inside the body. Studies show that different emotions can trigger the release of different chemicals in the body. For this reason, the hormone oxytocin has been nicknamed the "love hormone" or "cuddle hormone" because it is commonly released into the body when a person is experiencing specific feelings, such as love, bonding, and trust.[24,25]

However, in contrast, dopamine has been nicknamed the "reward hormone" because it is commonly associated with feelings of motivation, winning, and success. Unfortunately, dopamine can also be linked to negative behaviors, such as taking drugs, gambling, anger, and addiction because these activities can also trigger the reward center of the brain.[26,27]

From this research we can see the difference between the emotions that trigger the release of dopamine (reward and winning) versus the emotions that trigger the release of oxytocin (love and cuddling).

It is also well-documented that these biochemicals have the ability to support the health of the physical body in different ways. Oxytocin is known to help reduce blood pressure as well as increase pain thresholds, while dopamine can help support our motor control and movement.[28,29] In fact, research on patients with Parkinson's disease has revealed that the loss of dopamine-producing cells is linked to the development of symptoms of the disease.[30]

We could also compare these two biochemicals (dopamine and oxytocin) to cortisol, which is known as the body's "stress hormone" because, as the name indicates, it is released during stress. It also exerts different effects on the body. From this, we can see yet another way that different emotions can impact the body in different ways because they even trigger the release of very different biochemicals.

Additional research has emerged since my recovery in 2010 that provides further evidence to support this rationale. For example, in 2019, researchers found a link between lupus, childhood trauma, and PTSD.[31] The Lupus Foundation of America states, "Those who had experienced a high level of childhood abuse had a nearly threefold greater risk of developing lupus than those who reported the lowest level of abuse or no abuse."[32] Another study in 2020 found that the specific emotion of loneliness has been linked to an increased risk factor for type 2 diabetes.[33] Yet another study on police officers in 2022 found that different types of stress were associated with upper back pain versus lower back pain.[34]

In each of these cases, it is interesting to note there were distinctly different emotions connected to each specific illness. Yet it was clear that these reactions don't always take place when a particular emotion arises. For example, not every person will blush every time they feel embarrassed, and not everyone who feels lonely will get diabetes. Based on this research, it seemed that two things were true. First, emotions seem to need a certain level of intensity (consciously or subconsciously) to impact the body. If a person is feeling slightly embarrassed or has slight feelings of anxiety, this would not likely result in a physical response. However, if either of these emotions were intense, a physical response could occur.

Secondly, that there must be a certain mindset (set of negative emotions) connected with each illness. One way I was able to observe this concept was by again analyzing research on MPD/DID, which revealed that a person can have several alters (personalities), all of whom display stressful or negative emotions, while only some suffer from ailments. What stood out to me was that these were medically documented conditions and that the same ailments occurred with *consistency* in the same personality. For example, one personality might always suffer from back pain while a different personality consistently suffers from headaches.[35] From this it seemed that there must be a specific mindset (set of thoughts and emotions) that was associated with each type of illness.

GAINING A NEW PERSPECTIVE: MIND-BODY EMOTIONAL-ENERGY HEALING

Throughout six years of research, the topic of thoughts and emotions continued to surface. But each time they did, I thought to myself that the issue could not possibly be my emotions; it had to be more than that. However, no matter which way I looked at it, everything seemed to point at emotions as being the hidden yet not-well-understood culprit.

While our thoughts and emotions may be invisible, their impact is not. Above all, I just wanted to heal. As I pored over the collective research, I could see mounds of physical evidence that I just couldn't ignore.

- Stress has been associated with reduced immune function, increased cancer progression, and accelerated cellular aging.[36-38]

- A negative mindset has been linked to impaired healing, increased re-hospitalization rates, and prolonged recovery times even after surgery.[39–41]
- Stress can increase the production of free radicals in the body, which can affect the physical body in various ways. Furthermore, extensive research has established that there is a clear link between free radicals and a wide range of chronic diseases.[42]
- In rare cases, extreme stress can actually have fatal outcomes. For instance, there are conditions such as broken heart syndrome or situations where overwhelming fear can lead to a person being "scared to death."[43,44]
- Our thoughts and emotions can influence biophoton emission (light energy). Biophotons have been shown to support the basic functioning of our cells.
- Trauma can create physical changes in the brain. Furthermore, it's interesting to note that some physical illnesses can be diagnosed based on brain scans, such as multiple sclerosis and diabetes insipidus.[45]
- Our emotions can trigger the release of either positive or negative biochemicals, which can either help support our optimal health and wellness or wreak havoc on our bodies.
- Highly optimistic people can live up to 15 percent longer compared to those who are the least optimistic."[46,47]
- Optimism can speed up healing and postsurgical recovery times, as well as help protect against illness and death.[48]

… and more.

The more I opened my eyes, the more I saw just how much this evidence was all around me. In fact, I was amazed to find that the power of emotions was written about thousands of years ago in the Bible: "A cheerful heart is good medicine, but a crushed spirit dries up the bones" (Proverbs 17:22 NIV).

It seemed clear that by changing our thoughts and emotions, we could influence the physical body in a number of ways, such as through cell proliferation, biocommunication, and brain chemistry, which could then affect the body's health, either positively by promoting healing or negatively by potentially causing illness. It also seemed that, as it relates to illness, the part(s) of the body impacted depended on the specific thoughts and emotions.

DEVISING A PLAN FOR MIND-BODY EMOTIONAL-ENERGY HEALING

I decided to formulate a plan to see if I could figure out how to activate my body's ability to heal. I knew I would need to be very specific, since the effects of emotions are very specific. Since I'd already been spending four to six hours each day engaging in a combination of practices, including affirmations, chanting, giving gratitude, silent and guided meditations, and healing music, and mind reprogramming and release techniques, it was apparent that I needed to find a new approach.

I decided to simplify everything and focus on a few specific points that could theoretically activate my self-healing. This meant I needed to:

* Increase my levels of optimism and get new positive
  emotions programmed into my subconscious mind to
  maximize my body's rate of healing. Although I had
  always considered myself to be an optimist, I began to
  notice that I had underlying fears. Based on the research,

it seemed evident these fears could decrease my body's ability to heal

- Focus on amplifying my positive emotions. Since it seemed that intense emotions had the potential to have a greater and faster impact on the physical body, I started thinking about amplifying my positive emotions
- Work to identify the specific negative emotions that were stored, or programmed, in my subconscious mind and were therefore negatively affecting my body
- Free myself from any negative emotions so I could eradicate them from my subconscious mind
- Ensure that I made a genuine transformation so the emotional shift was a real and lasting.

Yearning to heal, I was excited to try it to see if it would work. I figured that if there were any other factors that I needed to change in my mind, they would reveal themselves to me along the way (which, thankfully, they did).

6

THE 5 FACTORS FOR GIFT MIND-BODY HEALING™

At the end of my suffering there was a door.

Louise Glück[1]

"Emotions are not logical." As I reminded myself of this well-known phrase, it seemed evident that if I approached emotions solely on the basis of traditional logic, then I would likely not be effective. In fact, it seemed I would need to acquire a different type of logic. After all, the subconscious mind doesn't store information, memories, and experiences based on logic. Instead, the subconscious mind is influenced primarily by two factors: *repetition* and *emotional intensity*.

For instance, children learning the alphabet can get this information programmed into their subconscious minds through *repetition* as well as emotions of positive feedback. A simple example of storing emotions in the subconscious mind based on intensity is to look closely at a couple's chosen wedding song, the one often played during the reception at the first dance. Because they are experiencing *intense* emotions while their special song is played, these two things (the song and the emotion-filled moment at their wedding) get linked together in their subconscious minds. This gets stored quickly in their mind without repetition due to their strong positive emotions. After that, every time they hear that song, even years later, it will remind them of their wedding day and the stored-up feelings will resurface.

From this, we can observe that information gets stored in a person's mind not based on logic, but simply because certain events happened at the same time coupled with a strong emotion. Therefore, they become linked together. That's it. If something negative were to occur with emotional intensity, that too can get stored in our subconscious mind. Not because we want it to, but because the role of the subconscious mind is to store information so that we can operate automatically and efficiently. This means that our subconscious does not question the information; it simply stores it and then it becomes part of our subconscious programming.

The problem is that since the subconscious mind does not rationalize information, emotions can get "miswired" in our minds. When this happens, the mind can inadvertently link up a negative behavior to positive emotions. One example of this can be observed with physical self-harm, such as a person who engages in cutting. In this case, unfortunately, their subconscious mind has erroneously linked up positive emotions—such as feelings of relief, euphoria, or control—to self-cutting. We can all have compassion for a person who is struggling with this situation; they did not *consciously* choose to link up these emotions in their mind.

Once a person gets information stored in their subconscious mind, it can continue to resurface automatically for the rest of their life unless they alter/reprogram the information in their mind. This is the reason a person can recall an emotional childhood memory at the age of ninety. And because our subconscious programming is automatic, we can find ourselves engaging in behavior or emotional patterns that we consciously deplore.

THE IMPORTANCE OF SUBTLE EMOTIONS

As I analyzed the subconscious mind to gain a deeper understanding, I once again reflected on Sigmund Freud's work. He so brilliantly documented how he was able to help his patients change the emotions that were buried in their subconscious minds, resulting in radical psychological transformations. Essentially, my goal was to do the same thing except I wanted to change the specific emotions that would enable my physical body to heal itself. Of course this meant that I needed to access information in my subconscious mind. I will share with you in detail about how I did this in the upcoming chapters, but one extremely important insight from this was realizing the importance of *subtle* emotions.

I could somewhat recognize that I had subtle fears lurking in the back of my mind, but I thought that they were no big deal because they felt faint and elusive. However, as I began to understand the subconscious mind in an entirely new way, I had an epiphany. I realized I had been thinking, *This emotion is subtle and illogical; therefore it can't be important.* However, as I gained a deeper level of understanding I instead began to conclude, *This emotion is subtle and illogical, and it has come into my mind before.*

73

Therefore, these are clear signs that this feeling must be stored in my subconscious mind!

Changing my awareness to recognize the presence of subtle and seemingly illogical fears was the start of a profound shift in awareness for me. From that point on, I stopped ignoring and overlooking the very emotions that were unknowingly affecting me in more ways than I'd realized. I share this with you because almost every human being does this very thing.

FINDING DEEP AND HIDDEN NEGATIVE EMOTIONS

I didn't know which specific negative emotions were hidden in my subconscious and preventing my body from healing, so I began to create a process to figure it out, which I will share with you in the upcoming chapters. As I was working through the process, I was surprised to find a buried feeling related to a traumatic event in my adult life.

Discovering My Negative Emotions Related to 9/11

Prior to my fall, I had worked for a global telecommunications company, testing and troubleshooting large communication networks. My work schedule was from 5:00 a.m. to 2:00 p.m. in California. On the morning of September 11, 2001, I was in my office in California talking on the phone with my coworker, who was in the World Trade Center in New York. My clock read 5:46 a.m. In New York, it was 8:46 in the morning.

Suddenly, I heard a loud crashing sound. Then I heard chaos and screaming.

My coworker screamed, "Help me!"

Then the phone went dead.

I called him back, but the phone kept ringing.

Not knowing what was happening, I sat at my desk, confused, trying to figure out what to do. When I looked up at the television monitors mounted on every pillar throughout the building, they were all simultaneously broadcasting a live video of the North Tower of the World Trade Center with smoke pouring from a hole on the side of the building.

My coworkers and I watched the breaking news in shock and confusion. Apparently, a commercial jet airliner had crashed into the building. That was all anyone knew.

About fifteen minutes later, at 6:03 a.m., we watched in horror as a second jet airliner approached and flew directly into the South Tower. With a gut-wrenching feeling, I suddenly realized what had happened to the colleague who I had just been speaking to. Everything inside me wanted to help him and everyone else inside the building, but there was nothing I could do. I felt completely helpless, like many Americans. By 7:30 a.m. California time, both towers had collapsed. I sat in my office in shock.

The company I worked for had a significant amount of telecommunication equipment inside the Twin Towers. When they collapsed, our network went down, which also served as the backbone for smaller telecommunication companies. That day more than ever, people needed to connect with their loved ones and colleagues, so I set my personal emotions aside and got to work. My goal was to help get services rerouted, if it was even possible.

Like most people during this time, I mourned for those who had lost their lives and for those who were impacted, and I honored the heroes. In the days that followed, I worked extra hours and did my best to support the people who were affected by the network outages. As I worked, I was surrounded by televisions continuously replaying footage of the attacks with repeating broadcasts of whether our national terrorist threat level was orange or red. While I felt grief-stricken for others, I had always been extremely emotionally resilient, so I continued to work. What I didn't realize at the time was that while I was working, emotions were being stored in my subconscious mind.

However, once I began evaluating my feelings for self-healing, I noticed there were two main negative emotions buried in my subconscious mind: 1) a subtle fear that I was going to die, and 2) a heroic urge whispering that it would be noble to die in order to save others. Although I knew that neither of these made logical sense, as I wasn't even in New York at the time of the tragedy, the emotions were still there.

As I came to understand that these subtle, illogical emotions could have a lot more influence over even my strongest conscious thoughts, I began to look more closely at how they might be affecting me. I also began to follow the "emotional breadcrumbs," asking myself many questions, including how often I had experienced these feelings and when they first began.

THINKING IN TERMS OF PATTERNS

In the field of psychology, it's well-known that people have patterned ways of thinking and feeling that are stored, or programmed, in their subconscious mind. As such, a person may have an emotional pattern of getting angry or frustrated.

Because these patterns happen automatically, a person may not even consciously realize they have the pattern.

As Sigmund Freud documented in 1914, people tend to unconsciously repeat experiences that are similar to their past traumas, and they can even find themselves in similar distressing situations.[2] This phenomenon is commonly referred to as "repetition compulsion" (or reenactments), which is defined in the *Merriam-Webster Medical Dictionary* as "an irresistible tendency to repeat an emotional experience or to return to a previous psychological state."[3-6]

While patterns of repetition can occur in any area of our lives, many times they can be more visible when they are extreme. For example, someone who has an abusive parent may find that a pattern of abuse ends up emerging later in their adult life. This is so common that it has a technical term: *revictimization*.[7,8] Research shows that as many as 77 percent of people who had suffered from multiple types of abuse in their childhood also experience abuse as an adult.[9]

Whether the topic of abuse feels directly relevant to you or not, you can still glean from this data that despite our conscious desires, patterns really do unconsciously repeat in our lives. This may include patterns of feeling abused, unloved, criticized, rejected, hurt, victimized, or whatever else. Most people just don't realize that the problem stems from a pattern.

When it comes to the past, it's common for people to mistakenly believe that "the past is the past" and that old emotions somehow expire. Or that "time heals all wounds." But if that were true, no one would repeat any patterns from their childhood or experience pain from their past childhood wounding. The reality is that people unconsciously repeat patterns throughout their lives. Unfortunately, time doesn't heal all wounds; instead, it gives us time to bury our old emotions, get disconnected from them, and then mistakenly believe the old memory is resolved and therefore cannot be impacting us. I wondered, *did I have subconscious patterns that I'd buried? ... or patterns that were repeating?*

Discovering Buried Emotional Patterns from My Childhood

While considering these questions, I recalled there were several ways this emotional pattern had presented itself in my childhood. I'd often heard the story of my grandfather being drafted into WWII as a young man. He was shot while helping to save the lives of others and went on to receive medals for his bravery and sacrifice. I had great respect and admiration for him. Reflecting on the past, I realized that I had associated in my mind that the most honorable thing I could do was to sacrifice my life to save others. I also admired that quality in several other key figures, including Martin Luther King Jr., Gandhi, Winston Churchill, and Jesus. I was raised in the Christian faith, and as a child I regularly went to church where I listened to sermons about Jesus' sacrifice for others. The more I thought about it, the more I recalled countless times, with the most honorable of intentions, that I said or thought that would die for others.

As I reflected with even more clarity, I could see another incident that had definitely impacted me. I had left town for a short getaway. Shortly after I checked into my hotel room, I heard a distinct sound, like fireworks or gunshots. As I looked out of my fourth-floor hotel room window, it became clear it was gunshots. Everyone was running for their lives. From my window, I noticed a young child, seemingly lost, standing in the middle of the street. I recall thinking that it would be noble to die to save him, although it wouldn't have been physically possible. Thankfully, someone else managed to scoop him up, and both emerged unharmed.

Although I didn't realize it at the time of the event, I began to see that my reaction was a patterned way of thinking and feeling rather than a one-off thing. Not only did I view it as honorable to be willing to die for another, but some part of me *wanted* to die, as though doing so would be the noble thing to do. I even felt that *not* sacrificing my life would mean that I was selfish.

There was another important piece of the puzzle that I recalled, which began in my childhood. When I was six years old, I was playing with several children, and one of the kids asked if I would die to save a loved one. Perplexed, I answered, "No." At such a young age, it seemed like an odd question to me, and not one that I fully understood—at first. However, after I'd answered no, the older child sitting next to me answered a resounding, "Yes." She would die for others. It was in that moment that I felt flooded with embarrassment and shame for saying no. I suddenly felt that my answer was somehow inferior and selfish and that my friend's response was superior, and it was what any good person would do.

The more I could see the pattern, the more I realized that while the events of September 11 may have intensified the pattern, it had been ongoing in my life in subtle, seemingly insignificant ways.

Once I became consciously aware of it, I could see that my errored mind programming had created two opposing emotions. One part of my mind had a growing fear of death while the other part *wanted* to die to save others, as though it would somehow allow me to gain back respect from that moment in my childhood.

Yes, this was nonsensical; it was as if one part of my mind was programmed to be excited to jump off a cliff while another part did *not* want to die and knew it would be extremely painful. And since it was part of my subconscious programming, my opposing thoughts were "triggering" subconscious feelings of fear.

RECOGNIZING THE IMPORTANCE OF A COMBINATION OF EMOTIONS

As I scrutinized every detail of the research, and began thinking in terms of combinations of emotions, I asked myself what other subconscious emotional patterns could be affecting me. I found that I had a strong feeling of survivor's guilt around 9/11. This translated into me feeling on a deep level that it was not okay to enjoy my life while others had lost theirs.

Upon reflection, I realized that my thinking was part of a bigger pattern. Growing up, I'd somehow linked up the belief that there were people who had no conscience and who did bad things. As a result, I had developed a belief that if I felt guilty, it meant that I was a good person who had a conscience. Conversely, if I had no guilt whatsoever, then it felt dangerous, as if I could suddenly not know right from wrong and thus start doing bad things. Therefore my feelings of guilt made me feel safe and as though I was a good person.

I knew this didn't make rational sense. Previously, I would have ignored such thoughts, but now I understood that these subtle, whispered thoughts were revealing my miswired/errored subconscious programming to me. After identifying these patterns, I knew I had to find a way to fully release them from my mind.

As I worked with my mind, I began to understand the reason that emotional patterns are so hard to get rid of, as well as how to effectively release them. I share this with you because after working with thousands of people to help them heal, I've identified a few important points you'll want to learn from my experience.

- Negative subconscious patterns can, and typically do, show up in both silly and painful ways without a person consciously realizing it. For example, a person may make comments that feel playful, such as laughing while telling a friend, "If I don't get in the car, my husband is going to leave without me." While she is laughing, she may also have an underlying, subconscious fear of abandonment that is affecting her health.

- Some negative subconscious emotions, such as feelings of self-sacrifice, self-criticism, or feeling a sense of pride in hardship, can feel like they are good or are helping you in some way. However, these emotions can affect your body's ability to heal.

- As we go through the upcoming process, you'll want to begin thinking in terms of emotional *patterns* in order to get lasting healing results. If I had only addressed the emotions surrounding the events of 9/11, I likely would not have healed fully because my patterned ways of thinking and feeling would still be presenting in other ways in my life.

- Even when you can consciously see that an ingrained emotional pattern is illogical, you still have to reprogram your subconscious mind in order to genuinely feel differently. In my case, this meant I needed to reprogram my mind with the belief that I didn't need to die for others in order to be a good or honorable person, and that wanting to die for others was ultimately a bad plan. Why not live and enjoy life with others instead? This was a much smarter plan!

MY RECOVERY

As I began to develop and apply new techniques to reprogram my mind, the changes started to influence my body and my pain reduced dramatically! I felt like I could breathe again. The healing wasn't perfect at first, but it was a great start. Some days were pain-free, while on other days the pain came jolting back. When this occurred, I realized that I still had more work to do to ensure the old emotional patterns were completely gone.

Through reprogramming my subconscious mind, I felt stronger and more capable every day. I began working on improving my balance and correcting my gait, and I started to move about freely without my wheelchair, walker, or cane.

I continued to modify my process until my body healed itself completely!

Soon I was able to join a gym and began working out to restore even more physical strength. After about four months of this, I felt well enough to take my first solo trip downtown, where I walked around without any assistance for the first time in years. Just me on my own two legs! It was pure joy and freedom. I looked at the city in wonder, soaking in the beauty of life: the vibrant blue sky; the tall buildings; everyone walking, talking, and laughing; the fresh air all around me. When lunchtime came, I watched droves of people pour out of the buildings to get food, and I felt like I was part of real life again. Awestruck that life felt so amazing, I walked around with tears streaming down my face.

I began reconnecting with friends and doing things like having lunches, dinners, and walks in the park. And as I regained more strength, I also began enjoying life to its fullest. I ran on the beach, played beach volleyball, and even began working on my pilot's license. The sky was the limit, both literally and figuratively.

I continued to follow through with the process for an extra two months after the pain had gone, just to make sure that my body fully healed and the issues did not return. And they didn't. There was no reoccurrence of pain nor of any other physical issues. And the freedom was blissful. I felt better than I had ever felt.

Looking back, what had started out as a desperate quest to heal myself ultimately turned into a spiritual journey to find myself and to understand life and human beings in a whole new way. I now call the experience a "spirit-full awakening," as my spirit felt (and still does feel) more alive than ever.

I was beyond excited to get back to living a full life in every way—enjoying time with friends and family, traveling, and also getting back to work because I loved my career. In preparation to return to work, I enrolled in school to study the many changes that had taken place in technology and telecommunications over the years I had been unwell, and to get a new certification for network technologies. I also began exploring ways that I might be able to share the process I used to heal myself with doctors and researchers, yet I didn't know of anyone personally. So I began my search to do that too!

But life ended up taking me in a different direction than I'd expected.

HELPING OTHERS HEAL THEMSELVES

People around me were amazed at my recovery, and as I began sharing my techniques with them, they too began healing from their ailments and injuries. Instead of going back into telecommunications as I'd planned, I began figuring out ways to help others. Since there was no traditional certification or school for the healing insights that I had discovered, I decided to get qualified in a whole range of healing approaches, from spiritual counseling to quantum healing and everything in between. Then I began working in a chiropractic office helping people heal themselves. As people began to reprogram their minds and fully embrace change, they were amazed by their results. They not only healed themselves but as they worked with their minds, they too found it to be an empowering and spiritual experience, leading to a renewed connection with life.

From there, everything continued to grow. My clients often referred their friends and family who then did the same. Before I knew it, I had a client waitlist and requests to speak at events.

While I was speaking on stage, I asked for volunteers from the audience who were experiencing physical pain. I would coach the volunteers on how to use their minds to free themselves from their physical pain on the spot. The volunteers were amazed—and so were the audiences!

At this point, I wanted to find a way to demonstrate the power of the mind so people could visually see its incredible healing power for themselves. I also wanted them to understand that the pain was not "all in their head" and that there were real physiological changes taking place. That's when I came up with a new idea: to use medical thermal imaging.

DEMONSTRATING PAIN RELIEF WITH MEDICAL THERMAL IMAGING

Illness and infection generates heat in the body. You may have witnessed this firsthand if you've ever sprained your ankle or had an infection and noticed heat radiating from this area of your body.

Medical thermal imaging is a high-tech, infrared camera that can capture an image of the heat that emanates from illness, inflammation, or pain.[10,11] In this way, it can help you to see where the pain or problem is in the body. If a thermal image was taken of neck pain, there would be a large red color on the image, which would show increased heat at the location of the pain or inflammation over the neck region. My goal was to show people their pain on the image and then watch it disappear using only the power of the mind.

I began searching for an expert in thermal imaging to work with, and in 2015, I found Dr. Hillary Smith, D.C., owner of Advanced Medical Thermography. She had owned and operated her chiropractic practice for over 35 years, which included thermography. Together we devised a plan and we were gratified to see that it worked even better than expected.

As people used their minds to release their pain, the image would change from red to green as their pain disappeared. Each person could clearly see that their pain relief was not merely "mind over matter"; there were actual *physiological* changes taking place in real time over the course of minutes.

For example, one volunteer had been suffering from neck pain that was at a self-reported level of 5 on a pain scale of 0 to 10. Dr. Smith took thermal images of the volunteer. On the images, the neck area was dark red which represented the pain she had reported. Then I began working with her, helping her to radically shift her negative emotions. As she did, her pain decreased from a level 5 ... to a 3 ... to a 2, and then it was gone!

At the same time, Dr. Smith and I watched as the images simultaneously changed from red to green. The volunteer did that herself by using the power of her own mind in less than twenty minutes. (If you'd like to see some of these images, you can find the images and video at brandygillmore.com.)

Every time I work with people to help them release their pain, I reinforce a few key aspects: 1) They were the ones who did it; I simply showed them how to master their own minds; and 2) They would now need to follow through to reinforce their new ways of thinking and feeling in order to achieve lasting results. Otherwise, if they reverted to their old ways of thinking and feeling, the pain could come back.

What is also interesting to note about this protocol is that Dr. Smith set her thermal imaging camera to automatically take a new image every second. This enabled us to watch the imaging in real time, second by second, as a person worked on releasing their own pain. From this, we were able to see negative results at times too. For example, if a volunteer *increased* their negative emotion, it would *increase* their pain and, simultaneously, the red area on the image would also *increase*. When I would say something to help them release the negative emotion, the volunteer would report their pain decreasing and the red would also disappear from the thermal images.

Since working with Dr. Smith, I have completed additional studies using a similar protocol, and each time the results have been consistent: as people have changed their mindsets and emotions, they have been able to release their own pain. This has demonstrated the power of the mind firsthand. At first blush, you might think it's just about relaxation or stress relief, but it's much more than that. To exemplify this point, I'll share the results from one of my other studies. Specifically, a small case study I conducted with Gaetan Chevalier, PhD, the research director of Psy-Tek Labs.[12] In this study, most of the volunteers had previously practiced positive thinking yet still experienced pain. Furthermore, one volunteer was experiencing a level 6 of neck pain. I coached him to use his own mind to free himself from his physical pain while he was being scanned using thermography. To his surprise, he was able to get his pain down to a 0, and the image reflected the changes: the area over his neck and upper back changed from red to green as his pain disappeared.

What is also interesting to note is that he'd just come from a ten-day healing and meditation retreat. Prior to the retreat, he'd attended a weeklong personal empowerment and positive mindset seminar. These therapies had done little to ease his pain.

My point in sharing this example with you is to emphasize that while these results may sound easy, they require a deep understanding of your mind and a level of precision. To help people achieve these radical results, I coach them to use their own mind to address at least one or more of the specific factors for GIFT Mind-Body Healing.

THE 5 FACTORS FOR GIFT
MIND-BODY HEALING

In working with people throughout the years, I have found that one of the keys to achieving radical healing results is to identify and address the *specific* emotional patterns that are associated with the health issue.

I also observed that there was never just one emotional pattern; there was always a combination. For example, a person who has a pattern of feeling angry may not suffer from a health issue, but if they also feel guilty, unsafe, or unloved, then that combination can be linked to illness and/or keep the body from healing. In some cases, a person may have three emotional patterns, while someone else may have eight or more. In short, the combination is always key. In total, I have found five categories of emotions that are associated with health issues and/or the body's ability or inability to heal (opposite).

I refer to these five factors as the "5 Factors for GIFT Mind-Body Healing." When you first review the 5 Factors, you may not initially resonate with any of the categories. This is because there's a high probability that you have hidden patterns you can't yet see, just as I couldn't initially see them in my own life.

The 5 Factors for GIFT Mind-Body Healing™

Factor 1: Positive Expectation and Optimism. Research has consistently shown that optimism plays an important role in optimizing your body's healing ability. To help activate self-healing, it's crucial to amplify feelings of Positive Expectation and Optimism.

Factor 2: Negative Punishment Programming (NPP)™. This includes negative patterns that can affect your health and hinder your healing. Examples include guilt, shame and self-criticism. This negative programming can impact you even if it is illogical, such as survivor's guilt.

Factor 3: Symptom Emotion. Each emotion has the potential to affect the body in a unique way. To heal yourself, it's important to identify and release the specific emotion(s) associated with your physical symptom(s). I refer to this as the Symptom Emotion.

Factor 4: Mind-Body-Soul-Spirit Needs (MBSS Needs)®. The body requires specific emotional-energy for optimal health, such as feelings of love, safety, and deserving. To heal yourself, it is important to ensure that these needs are met in healthy, positive ways.

Factor 5: Sense of Identity / Self-Image. Your mind has a blueprint of your self-image. If you've been ill, your mind may hold the identity of you being a "sick/injured person." That's why creating a positive, healthy self-image is crucial. Furthermore, it can increase your confidence and self-love.

Note: To the best of your ability, try to get adequate sleep and proper nutrition, including staying hydrated. This can support positive emotions and reduce agitation and irritability.

IMPORTANT NOTE: If you immediately notice a factor that applies to you, make sure *not* to dive right into it or into any negative emotions. In some cases, if you increase your negative emotions, you could simultaneously increase your pain or problem.

For this reason, throughout the process of self-healing, you will want to make a point to steer clear from going into your negative emotions. Instead, you'll want to make sure to start with the positive first. Then we will work to release the negative. As you will see in the coming pages, working with your mind in this way can help set you up for success and enable you to create a genuine change, which can turn into a life-changing GIFT. For that reason, I call the process "The GIFT Method."

PART TWO

THE 4-STEP GIFT METHOD

7

UNDERSTANDING
THE GIFT METHOD™

Every adversity has the seed of an equivalent or greater benefit.
—Napoleon Hill[1]

Welcome to a different way of working with your mind.

The approach I developed to help heal myself from my injury ended up being quite different and, in some ways, even opposite from the "norm." For this reason, I want to provide you with an overview of the GIFT Method so that you'll know what to expect ahead of time. This can help you avoid falling into old habits that might keep you stuck.

As the process unfolds, you'll learn techniques to help you reprogram your mind for self-healing. However, there will be certain parts of the GIFT Method that may initially seem counterintuitive. One of those counterintuitive parts is the *order* of the process.

Many people have developed habits of working with their mind in a particular order. For example, you may notice your mind wanting to immediately look for the problem. Or wanting to search for repressed emotions from your childhood. However, it will be important to avoid these common approaches because in doing so, you could inadvertently increase your negative emotions. As you'll recall from the last chapter when I discussed thermal imaging, when the volunteer increased their negative emotions, they correspondingly increased their pain. Based on this awareness alone, you won't want to "hang out" with your negative emotions during any part of this process.

This is part of the reason that it will be imperative to start the GIFT Method by programming strong, uplifting, positive emotions into your subconscious mind. Once you feel you have begun to feel them intensely, only then will you want work to identify and release the negative ones.

If at any point in the process you find yourself spending too much of your time focusing on your negative emotions, my suggestion is to take a break from the book until you are able to first focus on the positive before proceeding.

If you've been studying self-help or psychology for a long period of time, you might feel as though I'm asking you to avoid the negative altogether, or to engage in what is referred to in some communities as "spiritual bypassing," or "burying your head in the sand" instead of acknowledging or addressing the real issue(s). Please understand that the goal is by no means to avoid or bypass the problem. Instead, I'm asking you to implement what I refer to as Reverse Emotional Processing, which means processing your emotions in reverse order from the standard way by engaging only with positive emotions *first* before addressing negative emotions.

The GIFT Method was designed based on this reverse order. The four steps are:

- **Step G: Get** new healthy mind programming
- **Step I: Identify** the specific problems that can block your healing and affect your health
- **Step F: Free Yourself** from negative emotional energy and miswired mind programming connected to your illness
- **Step T: Transform** yourself by reprogramming and releasing unhealthy mind programming and then embody the transformation to get lasting results

Before you begin the process, there are a few key insights that can help you gain the clarity you'll need to get healing results as you work with your emotions. Additionally, these insights will help you understand the reason that processing your emotions in the reverse order, starting with the positive, is so important. You'll also come to understand why starting with the negative emotions will likely keep you stuck.

EMOTION-CONTROLLED PERCEPTION

Our emotions have the ability to shape our consciousness and the way we perceive, feel, and think about everything in our lives. This is what I refer to as "Emotion-Controlled Perception," and it occurs all around us, even if we don't realize it's happening.

One way this shows up in our world is through the expression "blinded by love," which means that a person is so intensely in love that they are unable to see or think clearly. In fact, research has shown that when a person is deeply in love (or in lust), they tend to see the other person not how they actually are but specifically through a positive lens—seeing only the good.[2-4]

Additionally, I have also found this can be true with negative emotions. If someone has intense negative emotions toward another person, their mind tends to see more of the negative in that person, or automatically "fault-find."

Have you ever experienced either of these in your life? Have you fallen in love with someone and could not stop thinking about the person? Maybe you even found yourself talking about them nonstop? In contrast, have you been upset or had an argument with someone and found yourself stewing about the issue for hours or even days? You may have even told yourself to just "let it go," but your mind continued going back to the problem. What's important to note from these examples is that your emotions are controlling your thoughts and your perspective.

If a person is living in a state of fear or frustration, they tend to notice and think about things that are fearful or frustrating to them. And if someone is feeling upbeat and happy, they tend to think of more things to make them happy. Likewise, our emotions (including our subconscious emotions) set the tone for our thoughts; they also control what we see and the circumstances we attract into our lives. The problem, though, is that our negative emotions can keep us locked into a cycle. This is what I refer to as the Emotion-Perception Cycle.

The easiest way to illustrate this cycle is to first start with the awareness that emotions get stored in our subconscious mind. For example, imagine a child who repeatedly experiences rejection. These negative emotions become stored in their subconscious mind and then attract repeated similar circumstances throughout their life. These stored-up, painful emotions begin to control their perspective, causing more of the same problems. Based on their life experiences, they develop beliefs about the world, others, and themselves, many times creating a negative self-image and low self-esteem. They may feel blame toward others and even develop defensive, aggressive, or reclusive behaviors that further perpetuate the problem. Each time the pattern repeats, new painful emotions are stored up. As you can see, it becomes a painful cycle that is hard to break free from.

Emotion-Controlled Perception

Subconscious emotions unwittingly shape our perception. This makes it hard to embrace a genuine transformation because we tend to believe what we perceive.

Subconscious Mind

Emotions and habits get stored in our subconscious minds.

Patterns Repeat

Repetition compulsion reveals that we can unknowingly repeat past traumas. Moreover, any emotion that is stored, whether it be positive or negative, has the potential to manifest as a recurring pattern.

Emotion-Perception Cycle™

(Aka The Emotion-Consciousness Cycle)

Subconscious Mind · Patterns Repeat · Unresourceful Mind · Unconscious Actions · Negative Expectation · Perception/Consciousness

Negative Expectation

After a negative experience, the mind may stay alert in anticipation that the problem may recur. This can ingrain negative expectations that further perpetuate the issue.

Unconscious Actions

Frequently, our actions, automatic responses, and subconscious behaviors unknowingly contribute to the perpetuation of the problem.

Unresourceful Mind

Negative emotions can cloud our minds, hindering clear thinking. This can prevent us from accessing new thoughts, perspectives, and ideas necessary for change.

Note: If you're familiar with my work, you may have heard me refer to this as the "Emotion-Consciousness Cycle." I use both terms interchangeably because emotions can influence our perception and consciousness. Also, each component can continue to influence any other without a specific order.

As you review this Emotion-Perception Cycle, there are a few things you will want to note as we go through the GIFT Method:

- This cycle can occur with any type of emotional pattern. From this you can see the reason why so many people get stuck in painful patterns that can affect their health, happiness, and lives.
- By starting with the positive, it can help you gain even more mental clarity to free yourself from negative patterns.
- The more you can stay in the positive, the better. This helps to minimize or avoid fueling any subconscious negative patterns that you may not yet realize are affecting your health.
- You can see the reason that working with childhood patterns first is not the best approach. After all, if your current mindset is unknowingly stuck in the negative emotion (and perception), then you will not be able to release it from your childhood self (who is also stuck in the same perception). As you'll recall, I had unconsciously felt that guilt and a desire to die for others made me a good person. Therefore to heal, I had to *rewire* my mind first, then *release* the negative pattern.
- Since we can see that our *emotions* control our perception, if you were to solely attempt to *think* positive thoughts, this would not easily shift your emotions and your perception, so likely you would fail to get results. For this reason, in Step G, there is an emphasis placed on creating strong, uplifting emotions to begin reprogramming your mind, thereby shifting your health and your perception.

When I mention bringing in positive emotions at the start of the GIFT Method, some people immediately think of gratitude as a quick go-to for positivity. However, you'll need to be much more specific than that to reprogram your mind.

Over the years I have witnessed many people who have tried to bring in feelings of gratitude in an effort to shift their mindset. However, because they also had underlying patterns that blocked them from doing so, such as patterns of guilt or feeling undeserving, they felt it impossible to connect with feelings of gratitude. This can be common and is something we'll address in the chapters ahead.

As we work through the GIFT Method, you'll find exercises to help you address this cycle, as well as each of the 5 Factors for GIFT Mind-Body Healing (from Chapter 6). For this reason, it's important not to skip any steps. The more you can follow through in a devoted and focused way, the more you will be setting yourself up for success. To provide you with clarity of the process, I want to share with you a quick, big-picture overview so you'll have a simplified idea of what to expect, making it even easier for you to implement in your life.

AN OVERVIEW OF THE GIFT HEALING METHOD IN ACTION: AIMEE

Aimee was referred to my class by one of her closest friends because she had a shoulder injury and was living in extreme pain. She had torn her rotator cuff and, according to her doctors, it would not heal on its own due to the type of tear; therefore surgery was her only option. However, when Aimee arrived for surgery, her pre-op blood work came back abnormal to such an extent that her doctors were uncomfortable and canceled her surgery.

Aimee was stuck without any other options. She tried her best to live with the pain but felt it was ruining her quality of life. She was unable to lift her arm, and on a pain scale of 0 to 10, it was often at a level 10. The pain kept her from sleeping and from doing the things she had loved the most in life. After all, she was used to being active.

She was a young grandmother in her early fifties who loved playing with children. She worked part-time at the local preschool, and when she wasn't working, she spent as much time as she could with her grandchildren. They lived in Florida and went to the beach as often as they could. Aimee was skeptical as to whether she could actually use her mind to heal her physical injury; however, she wanted more than anything to heal. Since she'd already tried everything she could think of, she decided to "give it a go."

Below is a quick summary of her experience:

Aimee, Step G: Get new healthy mind programming

During this step, Aimee worked on Factor 1 of the 5 Factors for GIFT Mind-Body Healing (Chapter 6), which was to genuinely raise her levels of Positive Expectation and Optimism.

When she had first learned about this factor, her initial thought was that she was already doing well in this area. She was known to people in her life as an optimist. However, Aimee was extremely motivated to heal, so she followed through with the various aspects of Step G and found herself surprised at how much lighter, more positive, and truly optimistic she started to feel. She genuinely felt more excitement about her life, resulting in decreased pain levels. The pain didn't fully go away, but it was a start. She was notably happier and started to laugh again with her grandchildren and the kids at her school. Her new, uplifted mind programming created a strong foundation for her to move forward with the rest of the GIFT Method.

Aimee, Step I: **Identify** the specific problems that can block your healing and affect your health

In this step, Aimee worked to Identify Factors 2 and 3 of the 5 Factors for GIFT Mind-Body Healing which are:

- Factor 2: Negative Punishment Programming (patterns such as guilt and feeling bad)
- Factor 3: the Symptom Emotion (the emotion that is connected to the specific ailment)

As Aimee went through the process to identify these two factors, she began to see that these emotions were connected to her marriage. Aimee's husband owned a construction company and frequently took on large projects in distant locations, often keeping him away for extended periods of time. As much as she tried to deny it to herself, the truth was that Aimee had been feeling lonely, hurt, and unloved. While he often gave her the option of traveling with him, she decided she'd rather stay home because she loved being surrounded by her lifelong friends, her children, and her grandchildren. She didn't want to miss watching them grow up.

Even though Aimee had met and married her husband knowing that he traveled for extended periods of time, she decided it just wasn't the life she wanted anymore. Once their grandchildren were born, her desires had changed. So while part of her logically knew it was not his fault, the other part of her was triggered and hurt.

Ultimately, Aimee found herself thinking and feeling like she was ready to "just leave him." She felt reactive, which was quite out of character for her, and she wanted to take everything with her, including their joint possessions and his things, too! That way, she'd be financially secure on her own. She'd been stewing on this plan for many months, and it had become more dominant in her mind as time passed.

Regarding Factor 2, Aimee was able to identify that she had guilt toward her children about wanting to leave her husband and therefore "break up" the family. She also identified additional Negative Punishment Programming (NPP), which was that in her plan to leave her husband, Aimee was justifying to herself that she could take whatever she wanted from their joint possessions. Until this point, she hadn't consciously realized that her actions were not in good integrity. Her angry emotions had been clouding her normal judgment to such an extent that she hadn't even realized she was justifying them. She was grateful for this awareness because she could now see that if she had followed through with her plan, it could likely have created a wedge between her and her children who loved their father very much, not to mention potential legal issues that could arise from it.

Regarding Factor 3, her Symptom Emotion: Aimee used the process described in the coming chapters to identify that her torn rotator cuff was connected to her feelings of wanting to literally "tear" herself away from her husband and her current situation.

Once she identified these negative feelings, she made a point to not "hang out" in her negative emotions. Instead, she turned her attention toward the positive and then continued on to the next step to begin freeing herself from the negativity.

Aimee, Step F: Free Yourself from negative emotional energy and miswired mind programming connected to your illness

In this step, Aimee used the GIFT Freedom Techniques to start reducing and releasing her negative emotions from Factors 2 and 3, which she'd identified in the last step. As she did, she felt lighter, freer, and had increased mental clarity.

Aimee moved on to the next part of this Step, which was to understand her MBSS Needs so that she could free herself from miswired mind programming and reprogram her mind at a deeper level.

Here is an oversimplified summary to provide you with a general overview.

- Aimee gained clarity on her Mind-Body-Soul-Spirit Needs (MBSS Needs), which are Factor 4. These include the need for love. She identified that she felt unloved by her husband and also began to see that she had miswired mind programming that was affecting her. As she began shifting these Needs, she further aligned her body with healing.
- After she identified the above issue, Aimee also noted that this had been a pattern from childhood that began with her father. He was always gone, and Aimee had felt unloved. Now she could see the same pattern playing out in her marriage. If you are new to the idea that our thoughts help create our lives, or repetition compulsion,

then it may seem outlandish that Aimee married a partner who was just like her dad. However, this tendency to repeat patterns is well-documented in developmental psychology where people often attract partners who resemble their parents or primary caregiver. Or, to put it another way, a relationship that recreates (in some respect) the same types of feelings and emotional patterns as those we experienced in childhood. This is referred to as Attachment Theory, created from the works of psychoanalyst John Bowlby in 1958.[5]

- If your mind is holding on to a pattern or hurt, there is always at least one reason for it. So in this step, to be able to free herself, Aimee began looking for miswired programming. As she did, she could see that her own mind *wanted* to hold on to the hurt. Her subconscious mind felt it kept her safe to remind her that men were not safe. (While Aimee had a few patterns, for simplicity, I only share this one with you as an example.) In short, she identified her patterns and the reasons they were miswired, and then she got excited to clear the longstanding pattern completely!

Aimee, Step T: Transform yourself by reprogramming and releasing unhealthy mind programming, then embody the transformation to get lasting results

In this final step, Aimee followed through to fully reprogram her mind using the tools and techniques I will share with you in the coming chapters. As she did, she was able to lift her arm fully and without pain! She continued to follow through so she could make sure the changes were programmed deep into her subconscious mind, enabling her body to heal itself.

She then began to upgrade her self-image (Factor 5). This is important because our minds hold an image of who we are, and if we have had an ongoing pattern around an emotional wound, it can affect our self-image. (Note: If you have been injured for any length of time, your mind may see yourself as being a person who is sick or injured, as though it's part of your identity. This is another reason it is important to change your self-image.)

Aimee realized that her self-image had become degraded over time. Going deeper, Aimee saw that she'd felt unloved by her father since childhood, and as a result, subconsciously saw herself as being undeserving of love. As she upgraded her self-image, she began to fall back in love with who she was again. (We'll discuss how to do this as we work through the process.) Aimee also embodied the transformation by following through with her actions which were to change her relationship with her husband.

Before explaining the rest of the steps Aimee took, I want to be clear that in most cases, I would recommend that people see how changing themselves affects the dynamics of their relationship before leaving it (assuming the relationship is not dangerous or abusive). This is because in most cases when people change themselves, the problem shifts, and their relationship tends to shift in a positive direction. While this may seem impossible, I have seen many people (even some married over fifty years) transform. As a result, their relationship improves, and they feel more in love with their spouse than ever. This occurs because a person's energy and actions can change.

An easy way to observe this change would be to consider the example of the pattern of rejection that we discussed in the Emotion-Perception Cycle. I mentioned that a person with the pattern of rejection may unconsciously engage in behavior that perpetuates the pattern, such as distancing themselves, being reactive, or being abrasive. In going through the GIFT Method, the goal is for a person to reprogram their mind and then embrace the change into their actions. This can transform a person's behavior and what they're attracting as well as the dynamics of their relationships. If you are in a troubled relationship, you may want to see if your changes help improve your relationship prior to exiting the relationship.

In Aimee's case, she was certain that she wanted a divorce, so I was not going to try to encourage her to do something she didn't want to do. Further, she and her husband wanted to live very different lives; he wanted to travel while she didn't. In her case, a divorce made sense.

By following through with Step T and changing herself, everything worked out even better than she'd hoped. She had a respectful discussion with her husband, and rather than leaving him without warning and attempting to take his belongings, they had an amicable divorce, which was healthy for everyone, including their kids.

Aimee and her ex-husband were able to continue co-parenting their children and grandchildren and have remained friends. Her husband (now ex-husband) had always made a comfortable income, and he was kind in the divorce. He paid spousal support and volunteered to financially help her open her own daycare center, which was something she'd always wanted to do. On top of it all, it was something she could do as a family business with one of her grown daughters. Aimee was ecstatic!

With no shoulder pain and full range of motion, Aimee was amazed that the GIFT Method had worked for her in so many ways! And so, too, were her doctors. They were in awe that her shoulder had healed itself. She celebrated with her children and grandchildren, and her level of happiness and fulfillment in life continued to grow.

Even after she healed, Aimee continued to use the GIFT Method to reinforce her new mind programming for another month—just to make sure that she *maintained* the changes rather than slipping back into any old, negative habits.

As of this writing, she has been free from her shoulder pain and is in a happy, healthy relationship with her new husband of four years.

As you may recall, Aimee could not undergo surgery due to issues with her blood work. However, after Aimee healed her shoulder, it just so happened that she was able to resolve her other health issues as well. As Aimee's life changed, her excitement grew to transform other aspects of her life as well.

That's also another important point you'll want to note from this example: Aimee addressed one issue at a time so as not to overwhelm herself. I would encourage you to do the same: address the health issue that feels the most urgent to you, then, once resolved, continue with any other issues. In many cases, by resolving one issue, you may simultaneously heal or improve others.

Now that you can see the big-picture overview, you can appreciate the importance of following each step in order. This approach can initiate a profound transformation in your emotional state, enabling you to shift your consciousness and break free from a negative Emotion-Perception Cycle. As you make these changes, it will be crucial to integrate them into your actions and identity. This is key to healing yourself and changing your life.

YOUR BODY IS GIVING YOU A MESSAGE

If someone had told me while I was in the depths of my injury that one day the very accident that felt like it took everything away from me would end up revealing to me a life-changing gift, I never would have believed it. But once I began to put the pieces together and learned to master my own mind, it didn't just heal my body; it changed my entire life in more ways than I could have imagined. And that is my hope for you. As you go through this book, I encourage you not to simply read it but to follow through and implement the simple but powerful tools and techniques. See what happens!

We've all heard the old adage, "Listen to your body." I have found that this is even more pertinent than we realize. I have come to view health issues as a spiritual "check engine" light on a car. It's as though pain and illness are trying to tell us that we need to stop and fix a pattern that's ruining our lives. When we do, it can be a life-changing gift.

Consider Aimee's situation: If she had gone with her initial desire to just "tear" away from her relationship in a way that was not in integrity, she could have experienced a lot of hurt and hardship. It could have severely fractured her relationship with her children and grandchildren and ultimately left her in a financial mess. Instead, she listened to her body and began to understand that, in short, her rotator cuff tear was a sign that she was trying to "tear" away from someone, and that it would be painful. So she changed her actions and her mindset and got clear on what she wanted. She was also able to free herself from a lifelong pattern of feeling unloved and now has a beautiful, loving relationship. By listening to her body and understanding that she needed to change, she turned the issue into a life-changing gift!

As you go through this book, I would encourage you to look at your life in the same way. Instead of thinking, *What else is wrong with me?*, work to understand the message that your body is giving you to change your patterns and, in turn, change your life.

Much like our innate ability to heal ourselves has been written about throughout history, so, too, has the power of our thoughts to influence our lives. Roman emperor Marcus Aurelius noted in his writings between AD 161 and 180 that "the universe is change; our life is what our thoughts make it."[6] While some people are well aware that our thoughts help create our lives, others dismiss this concept altogether as simply being an unfounded spiritual notion. Still many others remain skeptical because they have not yet been able to produce the results they desire. However, as you will see in the coming pages, in order to get real results, you must embrace real change. That will be your goal as you go through the GIFT Method: master your mind, transform your health, and change your life.

EXPANDING YOUR MIND

Another positive side effect of this self-healing process is that as you get more in tune with your energy and your emotions, you can begin to develop a deeper sense of intuition. I have seen this in some of my clients as well as in my own life.

If the idea that we can develop intuition is a new way of thinking for you, I understand. It may be helpful to recall that even Einstein spoke about the importance of intuition.[7]

He went so far to say, "It is intuition that improves the world, not just following the trodden path of thought," and, "Intuition, not intellect, is the 'open sesame' of yourself."[8]

It may also be helpful to take a few moments to observe some of the incredible and well-known ways that life communicates information in the natural world all around us. Birds know when to fly south for the winter and they know how to find their destination. Dogs have been able to use Earth's magnetic field as a compass to find their way home from hundreds of miles away. There is even evidence that animals can receive information that enables them to know when to evacuate prior to an earthquake. It's not that some animals can receive information from the world around us and others don't get the memo; all animals are uniquely tuned in to their own instincts. In the same way animals have the ability to receive this kind of intuitive guidance, I believe that all humans do too—including you.[9,10]

The way I now see intuition is similar to our ability to read and write. We all have the innate capability to read and write, but we must learn to develop the skills. The same is true with intuition; we all have the untapped potential. The more we clear our negative programming, the easier it becomes to access our intuition.

After I healed myself in 2010, my intuition began to expand. I found myself suddenly being able to feel what other people were feeling and knowing information that I couldn't otherwise have known. Since I had no prior experience of this kind of intuition, it felt weird to say the least, and I didn't want to tell anyone because I didn't wholly understand it myself. I am normally a very open person, but in this case, I assumed that since I didn't understand it, no one else would either.

Eventually, I shared my experience with Tina, a very close and dear friend.

A few days later, Tina happened to watch a segment on *60 Minutes* about a rare condition called mirror-touch synesthesia, a condition in which one person experiences the same feelings and sensations that another person is feeling. During the segment, journalist Miriam Weintraub was interviewing Richard Cytowic, M.D., about what she referred to as "almost this sixth sense."

I watched the interview and recognized that what I was experiencing was very similar in several ways. But in my case, there were also other pieces to consider, which I had trouble defining and weren't explained on *60 Minutes*. Not only could I feel what others were feeling, I also received information I couldn't have known previously.

I began to research this phenomenon and found several studies, some of which had even been sponsored by the United States CIA at the Stanford Research Institute in the early 1970s. In these studies, researchers documented a variety of abilities, including psychokinesis and remote viewing.[11] These practices sometimes went beyond lab experiments. For example, President Jimmy Carter once shared that the CIA worked with a psychic to help locate a missing United States aircraft when satellites couldn't find it. Carter has been quoted as saying that the psychic "went into a trance and gave some latitude and longitude figures. We focused our satellite cameras on that point and the plane was there."[12]

My point in sharing this information is to reinforce the fact that our minds are much more powerful than we give them credit for. And while many people may not take intuitive abilities seriously, they have been scientifically documented for many years, with research rapidly growing in this area.

I used to be one of those people who did not take intuition seriously; however, after my intuition and abilities unfolded, I began to understand intuition in a new way—as an energetic communication to which we all have access. For this reason, I began to refer to this ability to get information from the energy of the Universe as "Universal Wi-Fi." The way I see it, it's similar to the internet because we all have the ability to tap in and connect to this information that we call intuition.

For some people, this intuitive feeling may present itself as a strong gut feeling, while many others may start to experience chills/goose bumps, or they may have a sudden involuntary head nod. When I receive an intuitive thought or a message, the word "bingo" comes audibly with a thought or a message. For each person it can be unique.

As such, I would invite you to go through the GIFT Method with an open mind and be willing to connect with your own intuition. As you will soon see with even more clarity, our minds are truly incredible.

A FEW IMPORTANT NOTES BEFORE YOU BEGIN

1. It's important to support yourself with adequate water, sleep, and nutritious food as you go through the process. As you likely know, a lack of any of these can lead to feelings of irritability, which can make it harder to feel healthy and happy. That said, if there are reasons this isn't possible at the moment, please don't stress about it because that would be counterproductive. I've seen people go through my healing programs who have had health issues that made it nearly impossible for them to

eat solid foods at all or get adequate water. Yet as they worked through the process, they were able to resolve their issues and return to a normal, healthy diet. In any case, you'll want to discuss all changes with your licensed healthcare provider.

2. Be kind to yourself as you look for emotions and emotional patterns connected to your health issues. It's beneficial if you can simply view them as helpful messages from your body with an awareness that your body is trying to give you a "wake-up call" to make changes toward a better life. If you find something that you don't like, make sure not to berate or judge yourself; you didn't intentionally plant these negative emotional patterns into your mind. And the good news is, you can intentionally eradicate them.

Now is the exciting part: It's time to start the GIFT Method— to learn step by step how you can heal yourself and transform your life!

STEP G OF THE GIFT METHOD: GET

In this step we will focus on:

- Getting new healthy mind programming
- Creating your Power Vision
- Replacing Negative Moving Forward Visions
- Establishing new Positive Emotional Patterning™
- Techniques to amplify your emotional energy
- Factor 1 of the 5 Factors for GIFT Mind-Body Healing

This step includes:

Chapter 8
Get New Healthy Mind Programming

Chapter 9
Get Positive, Uplifting Emotional Energy

STEP G

8

GET NEW HEALTHY MIND PROGRAMMING

Imagination is more important than knowledge. For knowledge is limited, whereas imagination embraces the entire world, stimulating progress, giving birth to evolution.

—Albert Einstein[1]

It's common for me to work with people who are not new to the idea of self-healing. Many people who come to my classes and workshops have been stuck on their "healing journey" for ten years or longer, just as I had been stuck in my own life. If this applies to you, then likely you've heard about, and possibly even studied deeply, the topic of visualization. If so, then out of all the steps in this GIFT Method, the content from this first step may initially seem the most familiar to you because it contains guidance on creating what I refer to as a "Power Vision," which is similar to the practice of visualization. However, as you'll recall, during my injury, I spent time envisioning every day, but it didn't work to heal my body—that is, until I began to make some key distinctions. As such, you'll want to note the important details in this step, follow through fully, and do your best to turn it into a life-changing gift.

THE IMPORTANCE OF POWER VISIONS AND POSITIVE EMOTIONAL PATTERNS

A Power Vision is a vision for your life that is short, succinct, and to the point. A key distinction of a Power Vision is that the emphasis will not be on the vision itself but on amplifying your positive emotions. It's designed this way to help uplift your Emotion-Controlled Perception (the way that you see and feel about one or more areas of your life, and maybe even life itself). This structure is also important to help you begin establishing new emotional *patterns*.

If we take a closer look at the power emotional patterns have to influence our lives, we can consider the negative pattern in Aimee's life. As you'll recall, she had a subconscious pattern of feeling unloved, which began in her childhood with her father. Then she unknowingly entered into a marriage in which she also felt unloved. This painful emotional pattern, having been established at a young age, continued throughout her life.

Aimee's story is not unique; our minds are constantly attracting an array of repetitive experiences into our lives. These patterns can be positive and/or negative. In Aimee's situation, she had both. On a positive note, she had kids and grandchildren who loved her, which also resembled her upbringing; she had a loving relationship with her mom.

Knowing that our lives are heavily influenced by our subconscious emotional patterns, consider what would happen if you purposely programmed your mind with Positive Emotional Patterns, such as patterns of feeling loved, safe, confident, respected, happy, healthy, and attracting loving people. That is part of what we will be doing in this step: creating a Power Vision and then working to establish new Positive Emotional Patterns.

Once you establish new positive patterns, they can help uplift your happiness and your life because your mind can automatically begin acting on them, much in the way Aimee's pattern of feeling unloved repeated itself automatically. However, the key distinction here is that these are positive patterns that can attract more positive experiences into your life and make it easier for you to stay in emotional states that can support your body's natural ability to heal itself.

Part of the reason we'll be using a Power Vision to help establish new patterns is because visualizing can be an effective way to program new information into your subconscious mind. In fact, research has shown that our minds cannot tell the difference between a real experience and an imagined experience.[2-4] For this reason, we will be using a Power Vision to help "install" new positive *imagined experiences* into your mind.

As you get this new programming into your mind, it can help you create Positive Emotional Patterns as well as feelings of Positive Expectation and Optimism (Factor 1, p89), which can help lay the foundation for your healing.

ESTABLISHING NEW NEURAL PATHWAYS IN YOUR MIND

As you work through this step, it will be important for you to do more than just "think positively." Instead, you will need to think in terms of *reprogramming* your subconscious mind. To reprogram your mind, you will need to establish new paths (neural pathways) in your brain. These new paths can help you begin to automatically think, act, and feel differently. This will be crucial to your success.

A simple way to think about creating new "paths" in your brain is to imagine creating a new path in a field of grass. If you walk through a large field of tall grass and you take the same route over and over, a new path will be created in the grass. This path in the grass can make it easier to get to a new destination automatically and with ease. You'll want to use this same approach to establish new paths (new ways of thinking and feeling) in your brain.

The reason I emphasize this is because it's common for people to simply try to think positively about everything in their lives. While thinking positively is a good start, this won't typically be enough to create the type of new *paths* in your mind that will be necessary to heal yourself.

Continuing with the same metaphor, the approach of thinking positively in general (without having a focused plan) could be compared to walking through the field in a hundred new ways every day. This would *not* create new paths (programming) in your mind that you will need to succeed.

Let's continue to build on this metaphor in a way that can help you speed up your results: if you were to jump up and down along a grassy path, you'll be able to make a lasting imprint much faster! This would be akin to cultivating intense emotions with your mind programming. Strong emotions ingrain themselves into our minds much faster and deeper than regular thoughts. This is part of the reason that an intense, traumatic experience can become ingrained into a person's mind so quickly. However, in this case, you'll want to use this awareness to your benefit and be sure to amplify your positive emotions to establish positive programming more rapidly and create strong emotional energy.

A FEW THINGS TO WATCH OUT FOR WHEN CREATING YOUR POWER VISION

Over the years, I have noticed many people have outdated beliefs about self-healing that are keeping them stuck. In light of this, before you dive in to create your own Power Vision for healing, I will share a few common mistakes to watch out for so that you can set yourself up for success.

Don't Force Yourself

When it comes to formulating a vision for healing, many people mistakenly think they must create a vision to *convince* themselves they're already healed. I made this mistake during the first years after my injury, which ultimately kept me stuck. Perhaps this stems from the common misconception about the placebo effect: that it works solely due to belief. However, your goal here is not to force yourself but instead to work with the body's natural healing mechanism, which we can see is not dependent on conscious belief. For example, if a person has a scratch on their arm, whether they ignore the scratch or focus on believing it will heal, the healing process will still occur.

Your goal in this part of the process is not to convince yourself that you're healed. Instead, you want to focus on the power of Positive Expectation and Optimism to speed up the body's natural healing mechanism. As such, when creating your Power Vision, you will want to create a vision of what you do want and then simply allow yourself to enjoy your vision as much as possible so you can take in the positive emotions (and amplify the positive emotional energy)! As you follow through each day, it can help you establish genuine feelings of Positive Expectation and Optimism which can simultaneously start to decrease feelings of fear, insecurity, and stress in life.

A simple way to illustrate enjoying your vision versus forcing yourself to "believe" it, is to think about watching a feel-good movie. As you watch the movie, you're not trying to convince yourself that the movie is true; you are simply immersing yourself in the experience and allowing yourself to enjoy it. As you do, you may find yourself smiling while feeling uplifted and energized.

Similarly, you can think of your Power Vision as being a short, feel-good movie with you as the star. And since your brain cannot tell the difference between a real experience and an imagined one, the positive feelings you generate from your vision can begin to store up in your subconscious mind. For this reason, you will want to see yourself as being happy, loved, safe, healthy, and enjoying your life.

If seeing yourself as being healthy and happy sounds far-fetched to you, I understand. In my life, I wasn't certain that I was ever going to heal. Therefore creating a vision that included being happy and healthy didn't seem very realistic at first. Nonetheless, I knew that I needed to change my mindset, so I made a point to remind myself that all change starts from within. If you are feeling stuck, then I would encourage you to do the same.

Power Visions: Forward-Focused and with Integrity

Another common misconception about healing is that people believe their negative emotions originated from a past trauma, but that is not always the case. Emotions from the *past, present,* and/or *future* can affect the physical body.

I want to emphasize this point because if a person is unsure of what they want to include in their Power Vision, they might be tempted to skip this step. They may think that it's more beneficial to address their past wounds first and create their Power Vision at a later stage. However, this is a common mistake, which will not typically produce the healing results that you're wanting. Why? Because a Power Vision will provide you with an important foundation that is needed for you to genuinely begin shifting your mind and emotions *away* from any past negative patterns and toward what you do want.

Additionally, in most cases, the negative emotion(s) affecting a person are not solely connected to the past. For example, if we look again at Aimee's shoulder issue, we can see a long-standing pattern of feeling unloved by her husband that was active in her *present,* which was a pattern that originated from her *past* with her dad, which was also combined with a strong desire to abruptly leave her husband in the near *future.* She also had a fear of being unable to support herself. As you can see, Aimee was affected by a combination of past, present, and future emotions.

Getting a Power Vision was important for Aimee for another reason as well: She needed to make sure that her vision moving forward was in good integrity. That was a shift for her. As you'll recall, her initial intention had been to abruptly end her marriage and take everything from her husband. If she had kept this negative desire as part of her Power Vision, or continued to have this intention in any way, then instead of laying the foundation for her healing, it likely would have *blocked* her from healing. I've included an exercise in the pages that follow so you can double-check that you are on the right track.

In the GIFT Method, good integrity includes having *spiritual integrity*, which means not having negative desires to hurt, harm, cheat, deceive, or take from others in any way. This will be important for your own happiness and healing.

HOW TO FOCUS YOUR POWER VISION FOR HEALING

Prior to creating my first Power Vision, I had spent years working on various forms of visualization—even staring at anatomy books, trying to get the images "burned" into my brain that my physical body was healed. Despite doing this every day for years, my health never significantly improved.

Once I began to understand healing in a new way, I shifted my perspective. Thus my first Power Vision emerged. In this new vision, I stopped focusing directly on my anatomy and the physical aspects of my healing. Instead, I spent more time taking in how I wanted to *feel* while *indirectly* focusing on my health.

How did I do this? In order to focus *indirectly* on my health, I created a vision in which I saw myself actively playing beach volleyball. This was somewhat odd considering that playing volleyball had not previously been a desire of mine, nor had I played since I was a kid. However, since my goal was to picture myself being healthy without directly focusing on my injury or anatomy, I chose an active sport in an environment I loved.

Since I love the beach and being around people, beach volleyball became a simple and fun choice.

Specifically, I envisioned myself playing beach volleyball in the warm sun, listening to music, laughing and connecting with friends. In my vision it was a joyous, peaceful day. I imagined the sun, the blue-green ocean water, and the beautiful blue sky. I allowed myself to feel that life was joyful, happy, and safe. I programmed this vision into my mind each day while placing my focus on the specific emotions the scene aroused.

This vision came to fruition in a much different way than I could have expected. After healing myself, some of my friends asked me for help with their health, so I started sharing this information with them. One friend who had beautifully transformed herself and her life, wanted to thank me, so she surprised me with a first-class trip to Mexico to celebrate my healing and hers. What an incredible surprise!

It just so happened that when we arrived at the resort in Mexico, beach volleyball was being played right outside our window. Immediately, my friend suggested we join in even though she was not aware of my vision. In fact, after I'd healed, I had even forgotten about my vision because I was distracted by so many other exciting things. Yet through this completely unplanned and unexpected series of events, there I was on the sunny beach, feeling healthy, fit, happy, and carefree, playing volleyball with friends and listening to music. It didn't just feel like a game of volleyball; it felt like déjà vu. With happy tears in my eyes and a glowing smile, I savored every moment.

Prior to this Power Vision, I had never played or even been invited to play a game of volleyball in my adult life. To this day, I still receive wonderful, random invites to play from friends who have no idea about my Power Vision.

Over the years, I've personally experienced and also witnessed people's visions manifest through a series of "synchronicities" similar to my experience with volleyball. I've seen people create Power Visions to manifest the relationship they are wanting and, through a beautiful unfoldment, the relationship they envisioned manifests. I have seen the jobs people were envisioning come to fruition. This is one of the ways that self-healing can start to become life-changing because, in addition to helping to establish feelings of optimism, creating a Power Vision can also help direct both your mind and your actions to move toward your desires and help you create the life you are wanting!

Now let's work on creating *your* Power Vision.

Create Your Power Vision

As you create your Power Vision, you won't want to overthink it. When I created mine, I didn't know which specific emotions were affecting my body. I simply chose what I was craving inside. So, too, did Aimee. When she created her Power Vision, she was at the same stage as you are now: starting the GIFT Method and therefore unaware of which negative emotions were linked to her health. The vision she was pulled toward included the things she had been longing for. So your goal is not to feel stressed to create the "perfect" vision. Instead, focus specifically on creating a short vision that can help you shift your mindset and your emotions toward accessing more Positive Expectation and Optimism. Keep it simple and have fun with it. Below are guidelines to help you do so.

- **Get Clear on a Vision to Program into Your Mind.** You'll want to choose something that makes you feel optimistic about your life and your future. In Aimee's case, her vision was simple, yet it included all the things she was longing for in life, such as feeling loved, supported, respected, and financially safe.

Her vision was: *"I see myself walking around and smiling, feeling strong, confident, happy, and loved. People love me and are so nice to me. My ex-husband and I are very kind toward each other. This is working out nicely for everyone. I am making more than enough money to support myself, and it feels incredible. I am proud of my accomplishments and so, too, is my family. I am happy and healthy and feel strong in my body. Life is so great."*

- **Write Down Your Power Vision.** This can help you get the information into your subconscious mind. It can also help your vision remain consistent. As we discussed previously, it will be important to repeatedly "take the same path through the grass."

- **Focus on How Your Vision Makes You Really Feel.** Keep your vision simple so you can stay focused on creating and really feeling the emotional shifts you are seeking. Aimee's Power Vision is a great example of this. She made a point to include elements that felt loving, uplifting, and safe. This enabled her to read her vision and place her focus on these new emotions, so she could start to get these new emotions programmed into her subconscious mind. This began to shift her mindset and emotional patterns, which was key for helping her increase her Positive Expectation and Optimism in her life and for her future. You'll want to do the same; make sure your Power Vision is focused on how you want to feel to create change from the inside out.

- **Short Is Sweet: Don't Include Too Much** (less than one hundred words would be best). There's no need to include everything you've ever wanted in your first vision. Come up with something that feels good to help you establish feelings of Positive Expectation and Optimism as well as move your life in the direction you want to go. Then, after you achieve your first vision, you can always create another one, then another. Otherwise, if you include too much all at once, or if it doesn't seem at least somewhat realistic, it could backfire. Instead of creating positive emotions, you could inadvertently program in feelings of being overwhelmed or that it is impossible to change your life. For example, if Aimee had tried to picture herself as suddenly having ten million dollars, it's likely this could feel unrealistic to her since she had never experienced that amount of money before and didn't know anyone else who had. In this case, it would likely have been hard for her to conceive of and truly feel into the vision. Instead, she kept her vision more immediately tangible by focusing on her next goal and getting it into her mind. It still felt like a stretch for her at the time, but nonetheless a more realistic one. Then, as she began to imagine it each day, it became even more real to her. She continued to take action steps toward it, and it eventually manifested. That's what you'll want to do.

  Note: I'm not saying Aimee couldn't have ten million dollars. I've worked with people who had visions of taking their businesses to the next level who have achieved their vision and were able to make a lot more than ten million dollars. My point in saying this is just that I do not want to diminish or set limits as to what is possible for you if that is your goal. However, in Aimee's case, if she had set a Power

Vision that felt unrealistic and far from her current reality, then instead of helping her, it likely would have kept her stuck. The key is to stretch yourself with your vision and get yourself to feel optimistic about your future, without making your vision unrealistic. Then as you follow through and read your vision each day, embrace the excitement to take action in your life toward the vision you are wanting.

- **Avoid Focusing on What You Don't Want.** If Aimee had worded her vision as, "I don't want to feel unloved," then it would not have worked to help her bring in new positive emotions to create a strong sense of Positive Expectation and Optimism. From this you can see that it is important to keep your Power Vision focused on the positive and what you *do* want instead of focusing on what you *don't* want.

- **Set an Alarm and Stick to It!** It's important to set yourself up for success by establishing a routine. Start by setting an alarm and dedicating a few minutes each day to focus on your Power Vision. I recommend doing this at least twice a day, in the morning and evening, until your body has fully healed itself. During these sessions, let go of analytical thoughts and intentionally immerse yourself in intense positive emotions from your vision. By consistently repeating this practice, you can begin to program new Positive Emotional Patterns into your subconscious mind. Remember, the more you intensify the emotions derived from your vision, the greater the impact will be.

Check for Any Negative Moving-Forward Desires

If you have any negative moving-forward desires or intentions that are not in good integrity, they can block you from healing. For example, thinking about Aimee's Power Vision: If she had kept her initial plan to leave her husband and take his belongings, or if she had made her vision about finding another man to date prior to separating from her husband, these Power Visions would likely have backfired because they would not have been in good spiritual integrity. However, since Aimee stayed in good integrity and had an amicable divorce with her husband, it worked out in the best way for her and for everyone.

It's fun to note that even after Aimee healed, she continued to use these tools in her life. After she separated from her husband, she created a new Power Vision that included meeting a new partner. As mentioned, she is now happily remarried to a wonderful man who loves and respects her.

Now is the time to focus on your healing and examine if you have any negative desires in your Power Vision (or in your life). You may not have any, which is great, in which case you can skip this exercise. However, if you do have negative desires, you'll want to make a point not to judge yourself or feel bad about them; instead, take action to change them. Negative intentions can block you from both healing and bringing in positive emotions. Also, any negative emotion you're carrying around can easily become a pattern that attracts more of the same kind of negative situations into your life.

- **Review Your Power Vision.** Notice if you are trying to move forward in life in a way that is not in good integrity, either in your vision itself or in life in general. Examples may include:

- o   Desiring to hurt someone in return because they hurt you. For example: You feel that once you are healed you are going to get someone back (vengeful feelings)
- o   Planning to take something from others, whether money, creations, ideas, or possessions.

- **If You Identify Negative Desires, Replace Them with Positive Ones.** If you identify a negative desire, don't waste time feeling bad. Instead, simply modify your Power Vision to redirect and reprogram your thoughts and desires to align with integrity. Make it fun and focus on creating a better, happier life for yourself, just as Aimee did.

Get Clear on Your New Positive Emotional Patterns

Now that you have your Power Vision, it will be important for you to get even more detailed about how you want to feel so that you can create new Positive Emotional Patterns.

Positive Patterns are important for several reasons:

- When you establish patterned ways of thinking and feeling, it will be easier for you to feel lifted and stay in a state of Positive Expectation and Optimism, which will be crucial for your healing.

- As we discussed with repetition compulsion, our minds naturally repeat patterns. This means that, in order to change your health and your life, you will need to establish new Positive Emotional Patterning in this first step. This will help lay the foundation for you to free yourself from negative patterns in the coming steps.

- Previously, we discussed that emotions are more powerful than thoughts. Additionally, when it comes to visualization, emotions typically have an even greater impact than the vision itself. This may seem contrary to popular belief; however, if we consider Aimee's situation, her husband didn't physically resemble her father, yet the painful emotional pattern of feeling unloved from childhood unconsciously repeated itself. This observation highlights that when emotional patterns recur, they don't necessarily mirror past experiences visually; instead, they evoke the same feelings as before. This is the reason that as you focus on your Power Vision, you will want to place extra emphasis on your emotions.

- **Get Clarity on Two Specific Positive Emotional Patterns.** Choose two specific positive emotions from your Power Vision that you want to place additional emphasis on to turn into Positive Emotional Patterns.

  For example, Aimee had several emotions in her Power Vision: feeling secure, loved, safe, confident, strong, happy, and healthy. All of these were important for her to get into her mind each day, but it was also equally important for her to create new Positive Emotional Patterns, which is what she did in this step. She chose the two emotions of safety and feeling loved.

- **Write Down Your Chosen Positive Emotional Patterns.** After you decide on two, write them down with your Power Vision so that you can remain consistent.

- **Make a Point to Feel Your Positive Emotional Patterns.**
  Each time you read and feel your Power Vision, purposely
  bring your awareness to these two chosen emotions and feel
  them as intensely as you can. This can help you establish
  new Positive Emotional Patterns in your life.

Note: If you can't yet feel the new positive emotions with much
intensity, or at all, please don't worry. In the next chapter we
will be working through additional exercises that can help you
radically uplift your energy to get these positive emotions into
your subconscious mind.

Summary of the Key Exercises in This Chapter

- Create your Power Vision. Write it down, making it
  as clear, succinct, and uplifting as possible.
- Choose two specific Positive Emotional Patterns
  from your Power Vision and give them extra
  attention and emphasis each day to maximize their
  impact.
- Check for any negative moving-forward desires in
  your Power Vision.
- Make it a habit to read your Power Vision at least
  twice a day, immersing yourself in the emotions it
  evokes. Keep in mind that in order for your body to
  heal, you must change the way you *feel*.
- Set an alarm to establish a new routine to help
  ensure you follow through.

STEP G

9

GET POSITIVE, UPLIFTING
EMOTIONAL ENERGY

We carry with us the wonders we seek without us...

—Sir Thomas Browne[1]

Creating a strong, uplifting emotional shift at the start of the GIFT Method—as we began to do in Chapter 8—will be essential for self-healing. In most cases, the emotional shift needed to produce real healing results is *significantly* greater than most people think.

I mention this to emphasize the importance of following through with the tools in this step because in some cases people may think to themselves the same thought I had initially which was, *I'm already a positive person. I don't need more optimism.* However, even so, you will still need to lift your emotions to get results. As you'll recall from Part One, bringing in strong positive emotions can help trigger the release of "happy chemicals" in the brain which can further support both your happiness and health.

Additionally, it's common for people to get "stuck in their heads" and/or feel disconnected from their emotions and not realize it. When this occurs, you may end up only thinking about your emotions rather than feeling them. If that happens, then you will likely fail to get the results you seek.

For this reason, in this chapter I will provide you with two fun and uplifting techniques that you can use to amplify your new positive emotions so you can fully feel them throughout your body and nervous system and get them stored in your subconscious mind.

THE VISUAL REALITY TECHNIQUE™

The objective of the Visual Reality Technique is for you to align your body with your new positive emotions from your Power Vision so that you can *access* these emotions more easily.

What do I mean by "align your body" with your new emotions? Put simply: if your physical posture is not aligned with these new emotions or is opposite from them, then it becomes more difficult to access and program them into your mind. As a simple example, imagine a person is trying to program their mind with feelings of excitement or confidence; however, as they visualize, they are lying down in a deep state of relaxation. While feelings of relaxation can be nice, the feelings generated with their posture (relaxation) are opposite from the emotions they want to program into their mind (excitement or confidence), so it becomes hard or even impossible to access the new desired emotions. This may sound insignificant, but remember, our goal here is to work with specific emotions and to establish new patterns of emotions (to walk through the grass in the same way).

Further, it can be common practice for people to want to sit or lie down to try to "relax" while they visualize. In this case, they may *think* about their new positive emotions, but they are not typically able to *genuinely feel* them and amplify them.

To fully grasp just how much your posture and body movements can either block or help you access your emotions, try this exercise: Lie down and focus on relaxing your entire body as much as you can. Once you are relaxed, envision yourself being excited, feeling these emotions as much as possible. Notice how much you experience the feelings of excitement throughout your relaxed body and nervous system. Then, stand up (or sit up), smile, put your champion hands up in the air (or even move your hands with excitement on purpose), and try again to cultivate these feelings of excitement as much as possible. To the best of your ability, intentionally feel and amplify the feelings of excitement throughout your body!

Do you notice the difference in how the posture of your physical body matches—and reinforces—your feeling of positive emotions?

In short, the more you can move your body to align with the emotions you want to bring in, the more you can experience and amplify these new feelings you intend to feel. This can help you get out of your head and get the new emotions programmed into your nervous system to help speed up your results. The easiest way to illustrate the profound effects I have seen from this exercise is to share an example of a man from one of my courses named Eli.

VISUAL REALITY TECHNIQUE
IN ACTION: ELI

Eli suffered from multiple health issues, including extreme low back pain, which was the result of a horrible car accident eleven years prior to joining my online course. It had left him with severe injuries and multiple broken bones. After several years of treatments and physical therapy, Eli had partially recovered but was far from healed. He walked with a cane and suffered from extreme chronic back pain.

As Eli began working with the GIFT Method, he created a Power Vision and started working on his Positive Emotional Patterning. He chose two emotions: financial security and feeling supported. He chose these two emotions because for most of his life, he'd struggled with feeling financially stressed and unsupported, and lately, he felt both even more acutely.

Eli often found himself overwhelmed and feeling like he had to handle everything in his life on his own. Work, in particular, presented a significant challenge with an increasing workload, additional responsibilities, and minimal support from others.

To address these feelings in his Power Vision, Eli pictured himself being happy and healthy, feeling supported in life, and feeling financial relief and security. In his vision, he saw himself fully supported, working seamlessly as a team with coworkers, and confidently completing his workload. From this, Eli brought in feelings of financial security and saw himself feeling more at ease and more supported in life than ever.

As he followed through to reinforce his Power Vision multiple times each day, he began to notice very subtle changes. He started to feel a bit more hopeful in life and noticed small ways in which he felt more supported. Physically, his body started to relax just a bit. However, it was not much. When we discussed his situation during a Q and A class, it became clear that although he had great follow through, the reason he did not have a bigger shift in his emotions was because he was lying down while he was envisioning. I explained that in order to amplify his emotions, he could use the Visual Reality Technique. Since he had limited range of motion due to pain, I encouraged him to keep it simple and engage only in movements within his capabilities and that even small body movements were better than remaining completely still.

With that in mind, he worked on spreading his arms open wide while focusing on his vision, as if he was fully taking in the feelings that he was safe and feeling supported. He saw himself as being both a supported and supportive team member at work as well as feeling financially safe in life. He energized and amplified these emotions as much as he could.

The more he implemented the exercise with movement, the more he was able to cultivate and embody stronger emotions that he could feel in his body and nervous system. Each day he did his best. After about a week of working this program, he was well into making these new emotions strong and feeling them as much as he possibly could. Then, to his surprise, as he was implementing the technique, his pain level decreased! It went from a level 9 of pain to a level 3. This was the lowest it had been since before his accident. Eli was in awe.

While Eli's pain stayed at a level 3 for the remainder of the day, his results were not yet consistent. He was new to the process and experienced ups and downs. To achieve lasting results and free himself from pain completely, he needed to follow through with the rest of the steps in the GIFT Method to make these feelings his "new normal," which I'm pleased to say he did.

Eli has now been free of pain for over five years, and he feels happier, supported, and more confident than ever. Not only that, but when Eli's boss saw how well he was working with the team and the increased levels of productivity, he gave Eli a pay increase—and then several more as time went on. This was pivotal in every area of Eli's life.

This example illustrates that positive emotional shifts can start to produce healing results. With follow through we can manifest our Power Vision and create real changes in our lives. But to do so, the emotional shifts must be extremely *strong, consistent, and firmly ingrained.*

What's also worth noting is the way that Eli manifested these changes in his life. In some cases, when people hear the word "manifest" they immediately think that everything they are wanting is going to suddenly jump in their lap. And while windfalls can occur, they are definitely not the norm. Instead, what is most common is that as you focus on what you are wanting to manifest and then you genuinely shift the way that you think and feel, you begin to operate in a different way in life, consciously and/or subconsciously. This is when real change occurs. Whether it's in your relationships or business or in life in general, the more you change yourself the more you can change your life. So, as you implement this powerful yet simple technique, remember that your goal is not simply to go through the motions of these exercises, but to genuinely have a desire to embrace the change within you. This means allowing yourself to feel and think in a different way.

Implementing the Visual Reality Technique

A simple way to think about the Visual Reality Technique is that it's like much like virtual reality, except in this case you are using your own mind to imagine your personal vision all around you.

Another helpful way to think about this technique is that you are advancing your innate skills. If we look to the innate behavior of children, they wisely know how to have a tea party without any real teacups. We are all born with the power of imagination, but as we grow up, we mistakenly assume that it is a child's game instead of realizing that it is a powerful tool that can help us create a life filled with happiness and fulfillment. Your goal with Visual Reality is to take this innate skill to the next level.

To implement the Visual Reality Technique:

- **Imagine Your Power Vision.** Bring your Power Vision into your mind as if it's happening right now. It doesn't have to be a perfect vision with every detail worked out. As long as you have a vague gist of your vision, that's all you need. Thinking in terms of the tea party, you don't have to know the exact color of the cups as long as you can get a sense they are there. Your goal is to keep it simple and feel it!

  Using Aimee's Power Vision as an example, she could physically walk around with her shoulders back while making a point to feel safe and confident in her posture and movements. As she does, she could intentionally amplify these emotions as much as possible. Then, she could imagine family members acknowledging her accomplishments, then noticing how it really *feels* to receive their love, acknowledgment, and support. She could make small hand gestures or even simulate hugs or gestures of appreciation, then make a point to take in these feelings as fully as possible.

- **Use Your Physical Posture and Body Movement and Stay Grounded.** When you're working on your own vision, it's important to think of your vision in a grounded way so your vision doesn't feel "magical"; instead, it should feel like a wonderful part of your daily life. Keeping in mind that your brain can't tell the difference between a real experience and an imagined one, it's best to stay grounded and allow the vision to feel real.

  Let's say that your Power Vision includes going for a run, and this vision excites you and makes you feel strong, safe, free, and alive. To implement the Visual Reality Technique, you'd envision yourself going for your morning jog. Simultaneously, you could physically move your arms as though you were actually running, intentionally cultivating and amplifying the emotions of strength and freedom or feeling fit and alive as much as possible. If you can't move your arms, then maybe you could move your feet. Any movement in your body can be helpful, and you can do this even if you are sitting on the sofa or lying in bed.

  When I was injured and in extreme pain, every movement hurt. So when I implemented this technique, I started by moving just my hands each day (without moving my arms much) while I envisioned myself playing beach volleyball. Though it may sound odd, it helped me to access more of the emotions from my vision which, with practice, made my vision feel even more real. To this day, if I move my hands in the same way, that vision immediately jolts into my mind and my emotions. As you can see, your body movement doesn't have to be an exact match to your vision. The key is the feeling itself. Any form of physical movement, as long as you remain focused on your vision, has the potential to intensify your emotions.

If you think about it, we all know that body movement can amplify our emotions. Picture someone who is angry and motionless and then compare that vision to a person who is angry and waving their fists. We can observe that the simple act of waving one's fists could amplify the negative emotions.

Of course, in this case, you'll want to amplify positive emotions.

- **Physical Objects Can Help You Access More of Your Emotions.** If your Power Vision does not feel real to you, you may find that holding tangible objects that correspond with your Power Vision can make it even easier for you to generate and connect with the real, positive emotions. If your vision includes playing tennis, for example, you could hold a tennis ball as you imagine playing tennis. This can make your vision feel even more real and exciting, which will raise the intensity of the positive emotions you experience.

- **Smile While Inhabiting Your Power Vision.** Engaging your face in the technique will enhance the emotions that arise. Additionally, some research studies suggest that smiling can help trigger the release of happy chemicals in your body, help relieve stress, and can even be linked to increased longevity.[2] For this reason, be sure to smile throughout your day. Also, if possible, embrace any changes you notice in your posture, such as holding your shoulders with confidence. This can help you create a new norm.

- **Use the Visual Reality Technique Daily.** Each time you focus on your Power Vision, make sure that your body aligns with the emotions in your vision. Use this technique at least twice a day for thirty days, or until you heal yourself—whichever is longer. The more regularly and consistently you use it, the easier it will be to access your new positive emotions and create new "paths" in your brain which can help you get the healing results you want.

  If you are smiling and glowing after working with this technique, then you are well on track, so keep following through every day. If you are not there yet, that's okay. Keep doing the best you can, and work to improve your ability to connect with your positive emotions. As with any skill, it takes practice. With a genuine effort, as you follow through daily, it will become easier for you to access these new emotions.

  Additionally, there are other techniques in the GIFT Method that can help you make radical shifts as long as you keep following through and putting forth your best efforts. One of those other techniques is the Neuro-Transformational Music Technique.

THE NEURO-TRANSFORMATIONAL MUSIC TECHNIQUE™

A problem for many people who are suffering from a health issue or going through a challenging time is that it can be difficult to access new, positive emotions several times every day on demand to establish new paths (neural pathways) in the brain. Obviously if they can't access new, positive emotions, it's impossible to successfully program new information into the subconscious mind and nervous system. This was a challenge I had to overcome in order to heal myself.

There were times when I was low, to say the least, and I sometimes experienced moments in which I felt I no longer wanted to live. This may sound odd given that I simultaneously identified as an optimist. But I didn't identify as being depressed; instead I saw myself as being an optimist with an insurmountable problem. In hindsight, I was also depressed. And while Power Visions and the Visual Reality Technique were helpful of course, they were not enough. I knew that if I were going to succeed, I needed to figure out a way to "hack" the process and gain access to these new, positive emotions on a more consistent and repetitive basis so they could become my new norm. That's when I began developing a way of working with music that enabled me to access my emotions more effectively and quickly. This became what I now call the Neuro-Transformational Music Technique (for simplicity, I'll refer to it as the NT Music Technique).

If you've studied other healing modalities, then at first glance when you hear the word *music* in a healing context, you may immediately think of music for relaxation or meditation, or with special frequencies. This is certainly what I once thought, and I had been using all of those approaches for many years, but they hadn't worked to heal my body. So I decided to take the *opposite* approach, and instead of trying to get my body to relax, I decided to use the music strategically to help me do the three things I needed the most.

- **Access New Emotions.** First, I needed a way to *access* new positive emotions consistently and with intensity.

If you think about listening to music, it can make you feel a variety of different emotions very quickly, depending upon the song you choose. You can listen to a happy song and suddenly feel lifted or a love song and suddenly feel surrounded by love. Using this awareness strategically, I chose specific songs to help me repeatedly access the specific emotions that I wanted to program into my mind.

- **Store Information in the Subconscious Mind.** Second, it was clear that I needed to get these new emotions *stored* into my subconscious mind and nervous system so they could become new Positive Emotional Patterns. Fortunately, our minds are very adept at storing music and emotions together. As we discussed in Chapter 6, most people remember their wedding song without ever trying to do so because it gets stored in their subconscious mind with little to no conscious effort. I wanted to use this awareness to my advantage.

- **Increase "Happy Chemicals."** Lastly, I had been specifically seeking ways to trigger the release of more "happy chemicals," including endorphins, serotonin, or dopamine to see if they could provide any health benefits, such as helping to reduce my pain, improve my sleep, and help support my happiness.

  As I read through research on music, I found several studies revealing how music can help activate the reward centers of the brain, and that listening to music while experiencing *intense pleasure* can help increase dopamine.[3-6]

Based on these three insights, using music to reprogram my mind made logical sense because it could help speed up the process of shifting my emotions.

How the Neuro-Transformational Music Technique Worked for Me

When I began to work with this technique, I knew I needed to access Positive Expectation and Optimism (Factor 1); however, I genuinely didn't feel great about life. For this reason, my first *strategic* choice for a song was "Beautiful Day" by U2. I used this song to program into my mind the strong *feelings* that it was a beautiful day and that life was beautiful.

Every time I played the song, I didn't just listen to it as I would any normal song. Instead, I emotionally immersed myself in it so that there was no room for me to consciously think. I made a point to cultivate the most intense feelings inside me that I possibly could, embodying the feeling that life was indeed beautiful and safe. I decided to use this technique as the very first exercise in my morning, and then bring my Power Vision to mind while listening to the music (or afterward) because it helped me to create even stronger emotions.

Since I was at such a low point when I began using this technique, I knew that in order to make a radical shift, I had to do something drastic. I began to implement this exercise *every hour* to lift myself as high as I could. The more I did it, the easier it was to access the positive emotions. Initially, the positive feelings were just a pleasant boost to my day. However, like compound interest, as I persisted in practicing them each day and remaining consistent, they continued to grow and had an even greater impact.

As these intense feelings of Positive Expectation and Optimism (Factor 1) poured into my nervous system, it became easier to maintain my positive feelings. Each time I did this exercise, I would purposely set any thoughts aside and focus on nothing but the song, creating the strongest positive feelings that I could to the point that I felt as if I were glowing. If I ever did the exercise and did not successfully amplify my emotions, I would redo it until I felt like I had fully saturated my nervous system with these positive emotions. As I created a new, happy norm, I reduced my listens to six times per day, which was enough to ensure that I stayed lifted throughout the day while still working to continue to reprogram my mind for healing. I did this every day until I was completely healed.

As you read this, you may immediately think that you should build an entire "happy playlist." And while having a happy playlist *in addition* to this technique can be a useful asset throughout the day, it should not take the place of this specific and very strategic exercise. If you only use a happy playlist filled with several songs, likely you will fall short of the goal, which is to help you program your new Positive Emotional Patterns and new neural pathways into your brain.

When you do it correctly, the song will stick with you. To this day, if I listen to "Beautiful Day" it can easily induce happy tears and fill me with instant, uplifting joy because it is so intensely programmed into my subconscious mind.

Over the years, I have watched the profoundly positive impact that this technique can have on people who use it and follow through with it. Individuals struggling with depression have used this technique to create a radical shift in their mindset. I have seen this work wonders with people who have felt unloved their entire lives. By using this technique, they were able to strategically access and experience feelings of love for the very first time. As they followed through, these feelings became ingrained in their subconscious. Note: if the song you choose has a few words you don't fully align with, that's okay. Simply change them in your mind as you listen and focus on the positive feelings.

Even people who initially had doubts about this technique due to its apparent simplicity went on to have incredible breakthroughs with it.

THE NEURO-TRANSFORMATIONAL MUSIC TECHNIQUE IN ACTION: ROBERT

Robert initially felt skeptical that music could be taken seriously as a useful tool. A successful businessman, he found himself in a downward spiral from which he didn't know how to escape. He tried many anti-depressant drugs, but nothing helped. He had been diagnosed with serious prostate issues that made him feel powerless in life. Based on his level of outward achievement, no one would ever have guessed that he felt this way on the inside. When he came to me, he felt he was at his breaking point.

Since he was in such a bad place, I suggested that he try to avoid constantly *thinking* about his situation. Instead, I advised him to create his Power Vision and then add in the NT Music Technique each day so that he could start feeling the positive emotions from it, and programming them into his mind.

Robert chose the song "Eye of the Tiger" by Survivor. Every morning and several times throughout the day, he immersed himself in listening to this song. Each time he listened to it, he noticed as soon as the music played, he immediately felt empowered with feelings of strength and motivation. At first it was just a nice, uplifting addition to his day; he was definitely happier and he started to feel his strength again. Day after day, as he followed through, the emotions continued to build. He started to feel stronger and more confident to such an extent that one day he realized that he'd lifted himself and his mindset far beyond what they had been prior to his illness.

As Robert followed through with the rest of the steps in the GIFT Method, his pain and his prostate issue disappeared! Both he and his doctors were amazed.

Now it's your turn to try the exercise for yourself. Even if you are not in a negative place per se, the NT Music Technique can help you more effectively and more quickly reprogram your mind to take your health, your happiness, and your life to the next level.

Implementing the Neuro-Transformational Music Technique

While this technique is simple to implement, it does have specific instructions. As with anything, the more you put into it, the more you'll get out of it. Here are the guidelines for how to get the most from this technique:

- **Decide on One or Two Emotions.** Get clear on which emotions you want to program in. I'd recommend either choosing the emotions that you selected for your Positive Emotional Patterning in the last chapter or choosing an emotion to amplify the feeling of Positive Expectation and Optimism in general. If you are having a hard time feeling optimistic in life, I'd recommend the latter, which is why I used "Beautiful Day." That song helped me amplify my feelings of optimism toward life itself. I then continued on to use the NT Music Technique to amplify my Positive Emotional Patterns as well.

- **Choosing the *Right* Song(s) is Important.** Select one or two songs that can help you access and amplify the *specific* emotions that you chose. For example, if you've chosen to focus on feelings of love, you'll want to choose a song that helps you experience feelings of love, such as "It's Your Love" by Tim McGraw and Faith Hill. For feelings of empowerment, you could choose "Adventure of a Lifetime" by Coldplay or "Bigger" by Beyoncé. If you selected happiness in general, you could use "Happy" by Pharrell Williams, "Walking on Sunshine" by Katrina and the Waves, or "Sing a Happy Song" by the O'Jays.

- **Purposely Focus on the Feeling.** For this technique to work, you *must* be intentional with it. You'll want to think of this technique as an important mind exercise, not as though you are simply listening to a happy song. Keep in mind that you'll get out of this technique what you put into it. When you listen to your songs, make a point to set aside any stress and instead place your *undivided* attention on accessing and amplifying your specific emotions as much as you possibly can. For example, if you are focusing on bringing in happiness, don't think about everything that is going on in your life now. Instead, immerse your mind into the feelings the song generates and then work to purposely experience the positive emotions to the point where you make yourself feel euphoric. Focus on bringing in the feelings as though they have the power to create a radical shift in your life, because with *repetition, consistency,* and *intensity,* they do.

- **Consistency is Key.** It will be important for you to keep the same one or two songs for at least thirty days, listening to them at least four times per day, including first thing in the morning. If you're in a challenged mental space, you may want to listen more frequently—even every hour as I initially did.

If you are wondering how many times per day is right for you, this is how I gauged it for myself. I began by listening to "Beautiful Day" to get good at accessing the *feeling* from it that life was beautiful. Since I was new to the technique and I was not in a happy place when I began, I could sometimes access the emotions more readily than other times. If I ever did the exercise and did not fully feel the emotions or found my mind wandering at all, then I would redo the exercise just to ensure I was getting the information into my mind to my best ability. The more I followed through consistently, the easier it was to access the positive emotions. Like any skill, as I kept practicing, I became good at it and then it started to "stick." The easiest way to describe the feeling "sticking" is to imagine how you would feel if something wonderful happened in your morning, and, as a result, you felt a happy glow inside of you for the rest of the day. That's how I began to feel. Then I would listen to reinforce this feeling several times throughout the day. I was consistent and persistent and did this until the feeling became my new norm. I would recommend doing the same; get clear on the specific emotions you want to feel and then follow through however many times it takes to make these emotions your new norm.

- **Avoid Reinforcing Negative Mind Programming.** It's also important to avoid any songs that may reinforce your negative emotions. For example, if you've been feeling lonely, you'll want to steer clear of heartbreak songs. If you've been feeling sad, depressed, or shut down, make a point to avoid melancholic songs.

    During my injury, to my surprise, I discovered that I'd been inadvertently or passively listening to music that was reinforcing my negative programming. And it was not just that I, personally, was playing this music; it was even being played around me. One particular friend, Leah, helped me during my injury in countless ways. She even drove me to many of my doctor appointments, some of which were two hours away. It was common during the car ride for her to play some of her favorite music from the '80s, which included songs with lyrics about dying for others. Like a mantra, the song would get stuck in my head! I never thought twice about it until after I identified my emotions connected to 9/11 and the subconscious pattern of expecting to die/wanting to die for others. As I mentioned previously, once I identified the pattern, I could see that it had been all around me, even in silly ways, though I had never realized it.

You may be thinking, *But everyone listens to these songs.* And you're right. They do! The problem was *not* the song, nor was it my friend's fault for playing the song. It was my own errored mind programming. Since I had a patterned way of thinking, I processed the song in a different way than others might. Further, I would say that the occurrence of emotional patterns repeating themselves (repetition compulsion) doesn't only happen in big ways, but in small, subtle ways all around us.

I share this not to make you paranoid about what you listen to, but to say that if you are going to succeed at healing yourself, you must work to remove anything that is reinforcing your old negative emotions. Then give it your best effort to follow through to genuinely establish new, positive mind programming.

The techniques in this chapter can be pivotal, so you'll want to make sure to follow through. Once you feel that you can successfully implement these techniques, you'll want to keep going on to the next step.

In my work, I have found that your mind can block you in a few different ways from fully lifting yourself and healing yourself. The easiest way to think of this "block" would be to imagine a ceiling and that you'll only be able to lift yourself so high before you need to remove the ceiling. That's our goal in the next chapter: to identify and begin to remove any emotions blocking you from fully lifting and healing yourself.

Summary of the Key Exercises in This Chapter

- Use the Visual Reality Technique each day to amplify the emotional energy of your Power Vision and Positive Emotional Patterns.
- Use the Neuro-Transformational Music Technique several times each day to help you access your chosen emotions as often and as intensely as possible until you feel they have become your new normal way of feeling.

Note: Be sure to continue this positive programming from Step G (which includes Chapters 8 and 9) throughout the entire GIFT Method or until you have healed yourself, whichever is longer. In the following chapters, I will refer to these positive programming exercises collectively as the "Step G Techniques." These include your Power Vision, Positive Emotional Patterns, the Visual Reality Technique, and the NT Music Technique.

STEP I OF THE GIFT METHOD: IDENTIFY

In this step we will focus on:

- Identifying Negative Punishment Programming (NPP) that can block you from accessing positive emotions or from healing yourself

- Identifying the negative emotion that is connected to your health issue (the Symptom Emotion)

- Identifying Your 180° Shift (your new positive replacement)

- Factor 2 and Factor 3 of the 5 Factors for GIFT Mind-Body Healing

This step includes:

Chapter 10
Identify Patterns That Can Block You from Healing

Chapter 11
Identify the Message Your Body is Giving You

STEP I

10

IDENTIFY PATTERNS THAT CAN BLOCK YOU FROM HEALING

No work or love will flourish out of guilt, fear, or hollowness of heart, just as no valid plans for the future can be made by those who have no capacity for living now.

—Alan Watts[1]

Welcome to Step I. In this step, you'll be working to identify negative patterns that can block you from healing yourself. In some cases, these negative patterns can even block you from maintaining a positive mindset. For these reasons, it will be crucial for you to identify and eradicate them completely.

As you go through this step, you'll want to be as specific as possible at identifying problematic mind programming. If we were only working with our minds in a general way, we may never address the issues in our subconscious that are needed to activate the body's self-healing mechanism. Conversely, if we are specific with our mind reprogramming—clearly identifying the negative pattern or problems—this can help us to make real changes at a much faster rate.

In order to accomplish this, we will start by identifying any Negative Punishment Programming (Factor 2). Then we will implement a simple but powerful technique that can help you begin to reprogram subconscious NPP that may be affecting you.

HOW DOES NEGATIVE PUNISHMENT PROGRAMMING (NPP) IMPACT OUR LIVES?

Negative Punishment Programming includes any patterns—either emotional or behavioral—that for one reason or another, make us feel that we deserve some sort of punishment. Common NPP can include emotions such as self-criticism, guilt, shame, self-blame, or any behavior that makes you feel you are bad or deserve punishment.

These feelings can affect you even if they are subconscious and don't make logical sense. For example, I have worked with people who felt that they had hurt their ex's feelings when they ended a relationship. They stored feelings of guilt deep in their subconscious mind that made them feel as though they still needed to be punished even though it happened many years ago and they had stayed in good integrity throughout.

I have also worked with people who have had patterns of self-criticism, self-blame, or shame about a past mistake and struggled to effectively let go of the heavy feelings, or they simply buried them. Sometimes the mistake was minor or even completely illogical, such as those who felt guilty for being happy or having a good life while their friends and family were experiencing hardship. "Survivor's guilt" is another clear example of illogical programming. There is no logical reason that a person should feel guilty for surviving. But I have witnessed this pattern in people on many occasions (including within myself).

Another illogical example of NPP includes feelings connected to physical or sexual abuse. It's well-known in the field of psychology that a person who was abused can feel ongoing guilt, shame, or even self-blame even if they know, intellectually and logically, that there is no reason for them to feel this way. I note this specifically because I have worked with many people who have suffered from this issue and, as a result, these emotions were affecting their health.

In fact, research has shown there is a significantly higher prevalence of chronic health conditions among people who have experienced sexual assault compared to those who have not.[2] For this reason, if you have experienced any type of assault or abuse, it will be important for you to notice if you are experiencing any ongoing emotions from the trauma so that you are able to free yourself from the wounding once and for all.

NPP can affect people differently depending upon a person's subconscious beliefs about punishment. For example, one person may feel they deserve a harsh punishment for a minor infraction while another may have made a similar mistake and feel they deserve no punishment at all. As a result, a person who is subconsciously holding on to mild NPP might experience mild symptoms, such as a slight decrease in their daily energy. However, a person holding on to intense NPP may feel undeserving in life, which could manifest as a loss of appetite, pain, or illness.

I've also worked with people who were extremely hard on themselves and had very strict or punishing subconscious beliefs, so much so that they felt as though they no longer deserved to live. In some instances, this was linked to either life-threatening health issues or suicidal thoughts.

In any case, if you have emotional patterns of punishing yourself, or if you have uncovered stored-up feelings of punishment in your subconscious mind—even if you know these feelings don't make logical sense—then it will be imperative to begin shifting these feelings.

Before delving into the practical steps for identifying and releasing hidden NPP, it will be helpful to review an example to illustrate how it can affect both your health and your life.

AN EXAMPLE OF NPP IDENTIFICATION IN ACTION: SOFIA

I recently spoke at a conference focused on Complementary and Alternative Healing (CAM) modalities for medical professionals. After I finished the theoretical portion of my training, I wanted to demonstrate the profound healing ability of the mind. To do so, I asked for a volunteer who was currently experiencing physical pain.

A woman named Sofia raised her hand. She had pain in her ankle, which she rated as a 7 out of 10. She explained that it had started about four years earlier, and although she'd received several types of treatments, the pain persisted. Sofia explained that at the time she had injured her ankle, she had been feeling generally happy in life and didn't feel that she was enduring any major stresses. Because of this, she wasn't initially sure how the mind-body connection could be relevant to her for healing. (As you'll recall, I felt the same in my life. I share this because it is common.)

As I began working with her, we identified the problem: She had buried feelings of guilt from a "major" mistake that she'd made in the past. As a result, she felt as though she did not deserve future success. Although she was aware of these old emotions, she had not realized their potential impact on her physical health or success. After all, the mistake was in the past. However, these emotions were buried in her subconscious mind.

What she had previously understood about mind-body healing is that the emotions that affect one's health must be a type of trauma or major stress.

However, once Sofia was able to recognize this NPP, I then helped her to begin shifting her mindset regarding the issue (which you will learn how to do later in this chapter). In short order, she began to feel radically differently, and as she did, her ankle pain released. She was happily stunned, as was everyone else in the audience.

Although she had done a great job at shifting her mind, energy, and emotions and was able to release her pain in under fifteen minutes, I emphasized to her that in order to maintain the positive results, she would need to consistently reinforce these new positive feelings and also follow through with the rest of the GIFT steps. In doing so, she could completely eradicate the negative emotions from her subconscious mind. Otherwise, if the negative emotions were not completely gone, then likely the body would not heal itself, and the pain could come back.

A while later, Sofia emailed me expressing delight that the pain she had endured for so many years hadn't returned. As someone with a long career in healthcare, she was delighted to enhance her understanding of the power of the mind to heal, and was completely in awe to see that it really had worked for her.

I share this story to illustrate three key points:

- **The importance of *addressing* rather than suppressing NPP.** Although Sofia was aware that she had feelings of guilt from the past, she had been ignoring and suppressing those feelings.
- **The importance of identifying the *specific* negative emotions to help you get rapid results.** Prior to her experience with me, Sofia had been practicing mindfulness and had worked with several healing modalities for many years. But it was only when she addressed the specific emotions that were linked to her ankle problems that she released her pain.
- **The importance of creating a "moving-forward" vision.** The emotions that were blocking Sofia had to do with feelings from her past that were unconsciously affecting her feelings about what she felt she deserved moving forward in life. This is very common. For this reason, in the coming exercises we will be working to clear any NPP from the past as well as reinforcing feelings of permission to have a great life moving forward.

I understand that for many, this example may sound impossible. As you'll recall from Chapter 6, the reason I started demonstrating pain relief using medical thermal imaging is because I would not have believed it unless I experienced it firsthand. So I wanted people to witness with their own eyes this incredible ability that we all have. After all, we were raised our entire lives to believe this would be impossible. I can now imagine how people must have felt when they discovered we could sail around the world for the first time, or fly in an airplane, or when the first human being ran a mile in under four minutes. All of these things were considered to be impossible and even laughable at one time, and yet now they are our norm. If you haven't watched the thermography video or viewed some of the thermography images on my website, I encourage you to do so.

TWO TYPES OF NEGATIVE PUNISHMENT PROGRAMMING (NPP)

So far, the examples of NPP that we've discussed have been what I refer to as "internal" NPP. As the name suggests, this includes internalized emotions. However, it's also common for NPP to show up in more "external" ways through actions or behaviors that are not in good integrity.

In the following chart, you'll find a list of the most common internal and external NPP I have observed over the years. My hope is that this will be a good starting point to help you identify any NPP that may be unknowingly affecting you. As you review the list, if anything resonates with you, don't judge or criticize yourself. Instead, simply write it down so that you can begin transforming the pattern as we go through the process.

Common Internal Negative Punishment Programming™	Common External Negative Punishment Programming™
• Feeling guilt or shame • Feeling like a "bad person" (even if you consciously know you're not) • Punishing or blaming yourself or others • Feeling like you're in trouble (even if there's no reason to feel this way) • Being self-crtitical (this is not always an audible voice, but a way of feeling about self) • Feeling a desire to get revenge (even if you tell yourself you would never do it)	• Being mean, rude, manipulative, passive-aggressive or speaking poorly about others • Cheating or lying • Trying to take from others (physical possessions, copying ideas, pirating content, etc.) • Trying to destroy others' relationships (child custody, unethical relationships, etc.) • Taking anger out on others or trying to control others • Unethical behavior with money or finances

NPP CAN BE TRICKY TO RECOGNIZE

NPP can be tricky to identify for a variety of reasons, with the most common being *acclimation*. In many cases, people have experienced negative emotions for so long that they are no longer consciously aware of them. This is rather like wearing something you are not used to, such as a necktie or a very high collared shirt. When you first put it on, it may feel foreign or even awkward. However, after a while you get used to it, and eventually you don't even feel it on your skin any longer. The same is true with negative emotions. At first we may feel heavy or uncomfortable from them, but then the feelings dissipate.

However, the negative emotions are not gone; we've just gotten used to them.

Another reason that it's sometimes tricky to recognize NPP, whether internal or external, is that people tend to unconsciously normalize or justify their behavior, so it doesn't always seem obvious when it comes to assessing what is not in good integrity. For example, a person may (consciously or subconsciously) feel as though they have a right to be angry or to punish others or seek revenge, in which case they may not realize that their behavior is wrong. Gossiping about others or speaking poorly about them can be damaging to their relationships, income, happiness, and life. From a spiritual perspective, if a person has a habit of breaking down, hurting, taking from, or in some way damaging others, this is not acting in good integrity. If you are participating in this kind of behavior, it can affect your health or block you from healing.

In some cases, I have worked with people who thought they were doing something good, but in truth, they were not in integrity. One man I worked with suffered from debilitating back pain and identified that his NPP was connected to his online business. His desire was to work online from home helping spiritual businesses that promote good causes. He began reading books in earnest and watching videos from a few thought leaders in marketing and then he began selling their content as though it was his own. It never even dawned on him that he was taking from the people who had invested time, money, and resources coming up with their ideas and developing the content.

Once he acknowledged the issue, he was able to resolve it more easily than he'd expected. He sought permission to use the thought leaders' content and also began pivoting his business. In doing so, he was even more successful and was able to heal his back pain.

It is surprisingly common for people who are doing great deeds for our world, such as helping rescue animals or making a contribution in some way, to end up justifying behavior that is not wholly in integrity. Unfortunately, the negative emotion can be a contributing factor to their health issues. If you are ever in question as to whether or not something is in good integrity, the key is to always think about "spiritual integrity." Ask yourself, *Are my actions harming, hurting, or taking anything from anyone?* As you'll recall from Aimee's story, when it comes to your health, your intentions matter too!

Before we begin the process to identify your NPP, I have a quick exercise to help you get in touch with your emotions. After all, NPP can be both subtle and illogical; therefore you'll want to notice what you are genuinely feeling so that if you have any of these underlying emotions, you can eradicate them from your subconscious mind.

The Emotion Contrast Technique

Did you know our senses can get fatigued? For instance, if you've ever had the experience of smelling one fragrance after another at a beauty counter, then you may know that it can soon become hard to tell the difference between the scents. This is due to what is known as sensory fatigue, or sensory adaptation, whereby, in short, you have decreased ability to distinguish the difference between scents. However, if a new, *contrasting* scent, such as coffee beans, is introduced, it provides a "reset," making it easier for you to distinguish between the fragrances. This is the reason you may have noticed coffee beans at some fragrance counters.

The same type of decreased perception can occur with any of your senses. And, if you simply *contrast* information, you can gain clear information very quickly. For example, imagine two similar looking shades of blue on either side of a room. Due to their distance apart, you can't tell if they are the same color or not. However, if you place the two shades of blue right next to each other (in order to contrast them), suddenly your senses have more clarity, and it becomes easy to see the color difference. Two music notes played at different times may be hard to distinguish; however, if they are played consecutively, it's easier to hear the difference. If you have been living in a certain climate for a long period of time and then travel to a location that is significantly hotter or colder, the contrast may feel jarring. From these examples, we see that we can gain clarity with *every* one of our senses if we use contrasting sensory information.

The same is true when you're working with your emotions. Because we can experience several different emotions throughout the day, and many of our emotions are buried in our subconscious mind, it can be challenging to identify what you're really feeling. I created the Emotion Contrast Technique for this very reason. Similar to the coffee beans, this technique can help provide you with a sensory reset (or contrast) to help you gain even more clarity. While this technique is simple and at times even silly, it's also extremely effective.

- **Ask Yourself About a Silly Feeling.** Choose a feeling that is completely foreign or outlandish to you—something you know you've never experienced. For example, you might ask yourself, "What did it feel like in the past to be a ninety-seven-year-old frog wearing a bikini?" Obviously, that's a silly question. But this is the point. The more outlandish or ridiculous, the better it is. Another question you could ask yourself is, "On a scale of 0 to 10, how much do I feel that I'm really a piece of pineapple?"

- **Take in the Contrasting Sensory Information.** Much like you must sniff the coffee beans to provide a reset, in this case you'll want to intentionally feel for this silly emotion inside yourself and from your past. It's safe to say that you'll not be able to locate the outlandish feeling if it never existed. As you feel for the emotion, you will notice that you simply cannot feel it at all. As you have the feeling that the emotion is not there, that is the actual reset.

- **Feel for the Negative Emotion.** After you've had the reset (contrast), notice if you can find the negative feeling. To do so, you can now simply ask yourself, "Can I find feelings of _____ [insert negative emotion] from my past?" Next, feel for the negative emotion. If you can find the feeling at all, any more than the outlandish feeling above, this means that it's stored in your subconscious mind, and you will want to eradicate it using the techniques ahead.

  This technique can be used anytime you feel you need to gain more clarity as you work to identify and/or release your negative emotions in the coming steps and throughout this book.

Identify Your NPP

Since NPP can have such a profound impact on our health, it will be important to identify if you have any buried in your subconscious mind. To do so, we will go through a short step-by-step process. If you notice that you have several *events* connected to NPP, don't worry! Keep in mind that we can have emotional patterns that repeat themselves. So if you've had a pattern of feeling guilty, then likely it has shown up numerous times.

Regarding my own injury, once I was able to clearly identify the feeling of survivor's guilt, I began to see that it had been a recurring pattern since my childhood. If you notice that you have a pattern that has played out many times over the years, even if it's illogical, simply write the pattern(s) down so you can transform them in the coming steps.

This process for identifying NPP includes steps for self-reflection and helps you notice signs to look for as well. It would be best to keep an open mind but, above all, *be kind to yourself.*

- **Review the NPP Chart.** Turn to the chart on p164 and review the patterns of both the internal and external NPP to see if any of them resonate with you.

- **Identify Your NPP.** If you noticed that you have one or more of the NPP listed, great self-awareness! You'll want to write it down so you can transform it. Note: If you identified your NPP and you feel certain that this is the only one you have, then you can skip ahead to the "Give Yourself Permission" exercise. However, if you feel that you might have multiple patterns, it's best to follow through with the rest of the steps for identifying your NPP.

- **Check for Hidden NPP.** If you did not identify any NPP, it's worth considering at this point that you may not have any. However, I have found that it is most common to have some type of hidden NPP, even if it is illogical. The problem is that NPP can be hard to identify. For that reason, I have included a simple questionnaire that can help you gain more clarity, as well as a list of the most common signs that I have found to be associated with NPP. They are:
  o Difficulty accessing or maintaining positive feelings
  o Feeling like your mind is stuck in patterns of worry or "brain fog"
  o Continuing to attract (and therefore experience) hardship or negative circumstances in your life
  o Self-sabotage patterns, such as being unable to step into happiness and success
  o Low feelings or depression, even if life circumstances are good
  o Feeling extremely drowsy or falling asleep anytime you visualize what you desire
  o In some cases, a worsening of pain or symptoms on days when you are happier, or flare-ups before an event you've been looking forward to.

- **Take the NPP Questionnaire.** If you have not yet identified any NPP, but you are experiencing any symptoms or signs that show you might have one lurking in your subconscious mind, then you can complete this simple questionnaire to hone in on what you are *really* feeling.
  Ask yourself the following:
  o On a scale of 0 to 10, how much do I feel that I should be punished from the past?
  o On a scale of 0 to 10, how much guilt or shame do I feel about the past?

o   On a scale of 0 to 10, how much do I feel that I deserve to have a healthy and happy life?

o   Do I feel critical of myself, or guilty, as though I am doing something bad?

o   Do I notice feelings of guilt for being happy? Do I feel guilty for being happy in general or only around a particular person?

- **Observe Your Subconscious Emotions.** Notice if you can feel any emotional connection to these questions in the current moment, in your past, or in your intentions for your future. Genuinely try to feel for the emotion, just as you did for the ninety-seven-year-old frog earlier. If you can feel the emotion in your system at all, any more than you could find the earlier "frog" feeling, then it means the negative emotion is there in your subconscious mind. In that case, you'll want to write it down so that you can start working to shift and release it.

- **Write Down Your Findings Without Being Self-Critical.** If you were able to identify NPP, the next step would be to notice whether it is part of a bigger pattern and then write it down so you can work to eradicate the emotions or pattern in the coming steps. If you notice behaviors that are not in good integrity, make sure not to be self-critical about them; that won't help. Instead, be *kind* to yourself and begin working to transform those behaviors.

Whether or not you've identified any NPP, it can be helpful to program into your mind each day that you are a good person who truly has permission to live a great life. This can help make it easier for you to bring in positive emotions and heal yourself. The following exercise will walk you through a simple technique that you can use to program this information into your subconscious mind.

Give Yourself Permission

When you become consciously aware of any NPP, it can be empowering because it's an important key to healing and for creating a better life, just as it was for Sofia. When I worked with Sofia, I had her generate feelings that she did deserve a great life moving forward, and then we began to clear her NPP from the past. You'll want to do the same, starting with the positive emotions.

- First, you'll want to make a point to start and end each day by generating the *feeling* that you do have permission to have a happy and healthy life. We all do. An easy way to do this would be to incorporate these feelings into your Step G Techniques. For example, you could make a point to notice in your Power Vision that you are a good person and that you do deserve a happy and healthy life.

- You could choose a song and use the NT Music Technique to generate and reinforce these emotions that you are good and deserve a happy life.

- Now that you are consciously aware of any NPP, you'll want to do your best to avoid going into any of these emotions until you can fully release them. For example, if you now see that you have a pattern of self-criticism or taking your anger out on others, then you will want to make a conscious effort to avoid going into the pattern as much as possible. Note: Even if you are able to avoid going into the NPP, it's still crucial to fully reprogram this pattern in the coming steps to ensure that you release it completely.

- If you've made mistakes in the past, it would also be good to bring in the feeling that you can trust yourself and you are free to let go of them. We *all* make mistakes at times. Instead of beating yourself up, place trust in yourself that you won't do similar things again, and take in the feelings that you give yourself permission to live a happy and healthy life.

Power Writing: Permission to Be Happy and Healthy

To further amplify your positive emotions so that you can get them programmed into your subconscious mind, we will use the technique of Power Writing. While this technique can be used to help you program any positive emotion into your subconscious mind, at this stage of the GIFT Method, you will want to use Power Writing to reinforce the feeling that you are a good person who has permission to live a great life.

- First, write down a specific positive statement that you want to support. Make sure it is not more than one or two sentences at most. In this case, since we are working with your NPP, you will want to ensure it includes that you are a good person who has permission to have a good life.

For example, you could write down one of the following:

- If you have made a mistake in the past and as a result have felt undeserving to have a great life, you could write:
  o *I now see that I have permission to enjoy a happy and healthy life. We all do.*

- If your NPP includes feelings of guilt, you could write:
  - o *I am a good person with a clear conscience. I have permission to have a happy, healthy life.*

- If you have been critical of yourself, you could write:
  - o *I am a good person. I have permission to have a great life and to be kind, loving, and supportive of myself.*

- Now write down a list of several reasons why that statement is true—at least five, but the more the better. You will want to make it specific to your NPP. For example, if your NPP was self-criticism, then you would include the reasons you have permission to live a happy, healthy life, including the sentiment of being kind to yourself. List as many reasons as you can. For example, if you feel bad about making a mistake and need to let it go, you could write:
  - o *Everyone makes mistakes. I should not hold on to mine. I am free to let my mistakes go and have permission to live a happy and healthy life today.*
  - o *I have permission to have a happy and healthy life because I am a kind and loving person.*
  - o *I have permission to have a happy and healthy life because I am no longer making the mistakes I made in the past.*
  - o *I have permission to have a happy and healthy life because I am a great person, and I want the best for myself as well as for others.*

- Once you've made this list, read it again and again each day. Feel into each of the statements as intensely as you can so that by the end you feel lifted and elated. Also, bring in your body movements and posture as we discussed with Visual Reality. Step into the feeling and truly feel it. If you wish, read the list out loud to intensify the feelings even further.

If you have heard of positive affirmations, you can think of this exercise as being somewhat similar. However, there is a key difference with Power Writing: your goal is to create and reinforce *several* connections in your mind as opposed to repeating the same statement over and over, as you might do with affirmations. That is the point of creating the list as described; you will want to bring in each supportive statement as strongly as you can, which ingrains these emotions deeper into your mind.

Next, it is important to begin freeing yourself from any NPP you have identified.

The Stress Interrupt and Freedom Technique (SIFT)™

If you've been able to identify any NPP, it will be important for you to begin reducing any emotional charge you feel around the issue(s). This is because negative emotions can make it hard for you to think clearly and they keep you stuck even if you don't realize it. The more you can begin to relieve your negative emotions (big or small), the easier it will be for you to create a radical shift in your emotions and in your health. The Stress Interrupt and Freedom Technique (SIFT) was created with this in mind.

As the name suggests, your goal is to begin interrupting your negative thoughts and emotions. An easy way to think about this technique is to first recall the metaphor we used for *creating* new neural pathways (p120), where you walked through a field of tall grass to create a path. In contrast, your goal with this technique will be the opposite: interrupt the paths in your mind that connect you to the negative emotion or memory.

To do this, first I will ask you to imagine that the problem is far away from you. Then I will ask you to picture silly objects between you and the problem. Doing so can help you start interrupting the path in your mind. This can help give you some "breathing room" from the problem so you can begin freeing yourself from the grips of the negative emotion.

As you implement this exercise, you'll want to use silly objects that are not real, such as a banana that is as tall as a seven-story building. While this is obviously a ridiculous thought, it's important for two reasons. First, it helps you create a lighthearted feeling. Second, you won't want to link up anything real in your mind. For these reasons, it's best to choose random items that are playful and unrealistic. As you do this, it can help you begin to interrupt the stress path in your mind. You can use this to begin to get some instant space and relief from your NPP or any other negative emotions that you may be experiencing.

- Begin by choosing the specific emotion you want to work with. This can be your NPP or, if you don't have any NPP, you can simply choose any issue that is bothering you. If you have multiple topics, you'll want to work with just one at a time and complete the process fully before working with another.

- Close your eyes and place your awareness on the problem you chose to work on. Picture this issue gradually moving away from you, shrinking in size as it travels, until it becomes a tiny speck in the distance—perhaps even on the other side of the world. The purpose here is to create a clear sense of distance between yourself and the source of stress. This can enable you to begin to gain space and experience feelings of temporary relief from the problem.

- Then you'll want to picture the number 1 halfway between you and the stressor (which is currently on the other side of the globe). As you imagine the number, you'll want to give it sensory qualities, such as a color, size, texture, or even scent. For example, you might picture the number 1 being blue, cold, and as tall as a building. You do not need to picture every detail perfectly; the important thing is simply to have a general feeling for, or essence of, the number.

- Next, picture the number 2 between you and your far-off stressor. For example, make it six stories tall and constructed of yellow roses that smell delightful.

- Now picture the number 3 and, once again, give the number a different look, feel, smell, and/or texture than the previous numbers. Maybe it's made of berries or snow. Maybe it's hot. Maybe it's furry. Again, remember that the images don't need to be precise. A basic *feeling* that there are numbers with different characteristics being placed between you and the object is all that is needed. The goal here is simply to engage different parts of your mind by adding sensory information to help you effectively interrupt the negative emotions connected to the problem.

- Continue the same process with the number 4, then 5, all the way up to 10 and 20, and so forth, until you no longer feel as charged by the emotion related to your stressor.

- Although this technique may not completely solve the issue, your objective is to begin to break free from negativity and start shifting your emotions. With this in mind, it would be best to embrace any feelings of relief and then reinforce your Step G Techniques (p154).

Note: You will want to make sure you have written down your NPP. The end goal is not to simply send these negative emotions to the other side of the globe and then avoid addressing them. Instead, we'll be working to release them more fully in the coming steps. However, at this point, it will be important to use this SIFT Technique (p175) to gain relief and increased mental clarity to help enable you to successfully reprogram your mind and shift your Emotion-Controlled Perception.

This technique alone may help to reduce or eliminate pain, give you emotional relief, or create a positive shift in your health. However, even if you are able to achieve noticeable changes, it will be crucial to follow through with the other steps in the GIFT Method for long-term results.

By calming your mind, emotions, and nervous system with this technique, it can make it easier for you to identify other troublesome emotions lurking within your subconscious mind, which is what we will be doing in the next chapter.

Metaphorically speaking, if your house is tidy, it is easier to find an item you are looking for. However, if you're looking for a specific item in the middle of a very messy house, it would likely be harder to find. The same holds true for subconscious emotions; the more you clear your mind, the easier it will be to identify these subtle emotions. Therefore, if you find yourself struggling with heavy emotions, it can be highly beneficial to utilize the SIFT Technique to address these emotions before moving on to the next chapter.

Summary of the Key Exercises in This Chapter

- Identify any NPP. Use the Emotion Contrast Technique to help with the identification process.
- Implement Power Writing to reinforce the feeling that you deserve a great life.
- Use the Stress Interrupt and Freedom Technique (SIFT) to begin freeing yourself and getting mental space from negative emotions.

11

IDENTIFY THE MESSAGE YOUR BODY IS GIVING YOU

One can never know why, but one must accept intuition as fact.
—Albert Einstein[1]

When I first began searching for a cure, I could never have imagined that my own mind possessed the incredible ability to heal my body. Nor could have I imagined it would ever turn into a life-changing gift. And yet both of these things were true.

Ultimately, my injury was a wake-up call that brought my awareness to a problem I didn't know I had. While I would never want to reexperience my injury, I would not take it back if I could because of the way that it woke me up to change myself and my life.

I invite you to approach this chapter with that same mindset, remaining open to receiving whatever information or wake-up call that your body might be giving you. Be willing to receive it with self-love and embrace change to create an even better life for yourself.

Although it may initially seem odd to think that our bodies could be giving us messages, the reality is that our bodies are constantly communicating with us. For example, we feel hunger pangs when we need to eat or thirst when we need to drink. We feel discomfort if our bodies get too cold or too hot. We feel tired when we need sleep. We receive messages of intuition or a "gut" feeling. If we take in the awareness that our bodies are giving us feedback on everything from food, water, body temperature, and sleep, it doesn't seem all that outlandish that our bodies would also give us feedback/messages when our subconscious emotions are off, especially considering that our thoughts and our emotions help create our lives. But many of us are just not accustomed to thinking of things in this way when it comes to our health. However, I would encourage you to take a moment to embrace this positive perspective so that your mind feels excited to receive these invaluable messages. It will be helpful for your healing and this upcoming process as you analyze the emotion(s) impacting your health.

I also want to emphasize the importance of not approaching this process as trying to figure out what's "wrong" with you or searching for a diagnosis. It is not the intention of this book to provide you with any type of medical diagnosis, nor do you want to find fault in yourself. Doing so can block your mind from accessing the information that can help you heal yourself.

THE IMPORTANCE OF FINDING YOUR SYMPTOM EMOTION

As you'll recall from Part One, *specific* emotions can affect *specific* parts of the physical body. For example, a feeling of embarrassment can cause facial blushing and feelings of anxiety can lead to a racing heart or panic attack. When I was working to heal myself, I was able to identify the specific emotions I'd buried toward the events of 9/11, which was a key factor for my healing.

Since my recovery, I've worked with thousands of people to help them identify the specific emotion linked to their particular health issue in order to free themselves from that emotion and heal themselves. I refer to this as the Symptom Emotion because it is the emotion directly linked to the symptom or ailment. This is Factor 3 of the 5 Factors for GIFT Mind-Body Healing.

Remember Aimee with the torn rotator cuff and Sofia with the ankle pain? In both cases, it was only when they were able to identify their Symptom Emotion that was linked to their ailment, as well as address their NPP, that they were able to make the necessary changes and heal themselves. As a result, both were also able to change their lives. After healing herself, Aimee found the loving relationship she had been wanting, and Sofia was able to free herself from guilt which helped her step into success and change her life in several positive ways.

In this chapter, your objective will be twofold: first, to identify your Symptom Emotion; and second, to begin redirecting your focus toward new positive programming rather than dwelling on the problem.

UNBLOCKING YOUR MIND

In the last chapter, we discussed the awareness that your mind can block you from healing yourself or bringing in positive emotions. Additionally, your mind can also block you from identifying specific information in your subconscious mind, including your Symptom Emotion. While this may sound strange that our minds would block us from valuable information, it can be quite common. It's well-known in psychology that if a person has experienced trauma, they may not be able to remember certain events around it. Some people can't remember parts of their childhood for this very reason.

Such mental blocking doesn't only occur with trauma. Our minds can block us in a variety of ways and for a variety of reasons. Another example of this phenomenon is known as "writer's block." It occurs when people experience a mental block and are unable to access the information they need to write. Similarly, I have noticed that mental blocks can arise when it comes to healing; if we are stressed, our minds can block us from accessing the information in our subconscious minds.

This is part of this reason I included the Stress Interrupt and Freedom Technique (SIFT) early in the GIFT Method (p175). If you're feeling in any way stressed in this moment, before you go any further it would be good to implement the SIFT Technique toward whatever may be causing you stress. Doing so can improve your overall mindset and enhance your mental clarity as you go through this process.

If, at any time, you feel negative or self-critical, then it would be best to pause and use the SIFT Technique to clear those emotions and return to self-kindness before proceeding with the process.

KEY INSIGHTS BEFORE YOU IDENTIFY YOUR SYMPTOM EMOTION

Before discovering more about how to identify your Symptom Emotion for yourself, there are a few important things to note:

Address One Symptom Emotion at a Time

Every ailment and every individual symptom can have a different Symptom Emotion associated with it. This means if you have multiple ailments or symptoms, you're going to have multiple Symptom Emotions. But I recommend only identifying and working with one at a time, just as Aimee did, so that you don't overwhelm yourself.

If you have multiple health issues, you'll want to work with the one you feel intuitively pulled toward working on, or the one that would be considered the more serious issue. In some cases, as people release the emotions connected to the more serious issue, it can have a domino effect and help reduce or even resolve other negative emotional patterns, which could bring relief to multiple symptoms simultaneously.

Recognize the Power of Subtle Emotions

Symptom Emotions can sometimes feel very subtle or distant because they can be deeply buried in the subconscious mind to such an extent that we don't think they matter. As you'll recall, this was the case for me.

If you feel somewhat out of touch with your emotions, or if you are ever unsure if you have a particular emotion buried in your subconscious mind that you cannot see, the Emotion Contrast Technique (p166) can be a useful tool for helping you increase your awareness of your hidden, subconscious emotions as you go through this chapter.

Mixed Emotions Can Still Impact Your Health

In our daily lives we often experience mixed emotions. For example, we can love a person yet simultaneously feel frustrated with them. When it comes to patterns, we can have patterns of feeling loved (just as Aimee did with her own mother, her grandchildren, and her children), and simultaneously have patterns of feeling unloved (as Aimee did with her father and her relationships with men, including her ex-husband).

Another common example of mixed emotions can be found around the topic of forgiveness. Many people mistakenly think that if you forgive someone, it will simply cancel out or replace the initial negative feeling of hurt or resentment. However, that is not the case. Instead, what you will typically end up with is a new feeling of forgiveness *as well as* the old feeling of hurt or resentment. Unfortunately, patterns such as these can continue to repeat in our lives until we fully eradicate them.

Here's a simple analogy for this: If you put a new sofa in your living room, it won't "cancel out" the old one. They will both exist until you take the time and effort to remove the old one. Similarly, when you're looking for your own Symptom Emotion, it will be important not to overlook any mixed emotions by thinking they don't count.

Don't Validate Negative Emotions

If you end up uncovering a painful story in the process of identifying your Symptom Emotion, it's important not to validate the feelings around this in any way. Instead, be willing to let go of the negative feelings in order to heal. Remember, if you increase your negative emotions, you could increase the issue. So instead of validating the negative story, you could use SIFT to begin getting some distance from it, then proceed through the rest of the GIFT steps to fully release it.

If at any time you find yourself validating negative emotions or criticizing yourself, then it would be good to take some time away from this book and proceed with the process when you are willing to be kind, loving, and wholly ready to support yourself with positivity. That is the mindset you will need to help you get clear on the message your body wants to give you.

TWO APPROACHES FOR IDENTIFYING YOUR SYMPTOM EMOTION

When I was searching for ways to heal after my injury, I began to consider my specific ailments and ask myself questions, such as: *What emotions could be affecting my physical body? If each emotion affects the body in a different way, how can I identify the specific emotion that is affecting me?*

Ultimately, this led me to develop two different ways to understand what my body was trying to tell me:

- A logical "Interpret the Ailment"™ approach to identifying Symptom Emotions
- An intuitive "Ask the Ailment"™ approach to identifying Symptom Emotions

As we review each of these methods, you may naturally feel pulled toward one approach over the other, which is great, and you may want to use that method first. However, I would encourage you to try both methods even if it's a bit of a stretch for you.

A LOGICAL APPROACH TO "INTERPRET THE AILMENT"

In Part One, I mentioned that I'd been studying metaphysics and everything I could find on the mind and energy. In doing so, I came across the work of Florence Scovel Shinn, a pioneer in the New Thought Movement in the early 1900s. In her work she taught that different health issues could have a different metaphysical meaning attached to them. This is what set me on the journey to begin noticing the various ways that different emotions could affect the body and our brain chemistry.

As I continued my research, I began to see the mind-body connection in a new way. It seemed that there was a logical connection between our emotions and the way they affected the body. For example, if a person was particularly stressed out about things they were hearing (in life, on the news, from friends, etc.), then they might have issues with their hearing.

Once I began to look at the body from this new perspective, this logic seemed obvious. Surprisingly, it was all around us! I began to notice it in our language and through common idioms. Even though it was always there, I hadn't seen it. For example, a person may experience something that makes them "sick to their stomach" or have "knots in their stomach" or makes their "head spin." Perhaps they feel that someone is a "pain in the neck" or a "pain in the rear" or "stabbing them in the back." In the coming pages, I will expand on this awareness because, surprisingly, these emotions can influence the health of the physical body.

With this awareness, I began to decipher which emotions were connected to specific parts of the body. In doing so, I discovered that the Symptom Emotion was typically connected to two things:

1. The *function* of the affected body part and/or ailment
2. The *emotions* associated with that function and/or dysfunction

With this understanding, you can analyze your health issues while keeping these two points in mind. For example, if you have an issue with your eyesight, you'd first notice the *function* of the eyes, which is to acquire visual information (seeing). Then you'd begin to observe any negative emotions that you may have toward that function (seeing) or the dysfunction (not seeing).

I've found that when people have eye-related issues, the body is often trying to tell them something about either what they *are seeing* or what they are *not wanting to see*. For example, I've worked with people who had a deep underlying fear or avoidance of looking at their bills or finances, or in some cases, people had a fear of looking at the future. Sometimes this can be felt so intensely that a person may even develop feelings that it is not safe to see. Or a person may be *seeing* aspects of life through a negative, fearful, distrusting, or critical lens. Another common emotion that I've found associated with the eyes is a feeling that "information is complex," so a person may feel they are secretly not smart or as though everything is "blurry," so to speak.

Over the years, I have worked with people who were able to correct issues with their vision by resolving these associated emotions. Given the widespread belief that poor eyesight is incurable, the idea that we can improve our vision through the power of our minds and emotions may seem implausible.

However, there are medical studies which conclude that stress can lead to a variety of issues with eyesight, some of which suggest that reducing stress can help restore eyesight.[2] Further, if we refer back to the research on MPD/DID, we know that when people switch between personalities (alters), they can experience significant differences in their eyesight.[3] We even briefly discussed the case study of the woman who was blind in some personalities but not in others.[4] This reveals the level of influence our minds can have over conditions that we believed to have been incurable.

Since I'd used the concept of embarrassment and facial blushing as a simple example throughout my research, I began to wonder why blushing related to the facial area. Using this logical interpretion approach, I asked, "What is the function of the face?" Its basic function is to socially connect with others; how they see us and how we express ourselves to them. Therefore the *emotions* associated with the face would be our feelings about how we express ourselves to others and how others see us. From this, it seemed logical to me that the emotion of embarrassment would show up on the face as opposed to any other part of the body. Why? Quite simply because embarrassment is a negative feeling about the way we are expressing ourselves or our feelings about how we assume that others are seeing us.

I've worked with people who suffered from atypical facial pain (AFP), which, as the name suggests, is chronic facial pain. In each instance, the Symptom Emotion that was connected to the pain was directly related to the person's feelings about how people saw them. For example, I have worked with people who felt strongly that others were judging their appearance, and in some cases, people were highly self-conscious or critical of their own appearance.

At times, it might be difficult to see the logic. As we have discussed, your mind can block you from seeing information in a new way. If this feels too far outside of the box, I encourage you to listen to my podcast episode where I worked with a woman to help her release her facial pain. Listening to her experience might help deepen your understanding of the mind-body-emotional connection, which will likely make it much easier for you to identify your own Symptom Emotion in the coming steps. (A link to this episode can be found on the website for this book.)

Identifying My Symptom Emotion

During the time I was injured, I applied this logical perspective to my own issues to identify my Symptom Emotion. To do so, I thought about complex regional pain syndrome (CRPS) in simplified terms as an abnormal or intense reaction or overreaction of the nervous system's function. Then I considered the primary functions of the nervous system: communicating information throughout the body; playing a vital role in nearly everything we do, from breathing to walking; and helping us react to stimuli. As I thought about how and why the nervous system reacts, I also contemplated the body's fear response, often referred to as "fight, flight, or freeze." As a result, I started asking myself questions: *Do I have an abnormal desire to fight, flight, or freeze? What emotion could be causing my nervous system to have an "abnormal" painful reaction? What event or emotion could make my nervous system want to overreact? Is there something or someone "getting on my nerves"?*

When I pondered these questions, the answers that surfaced led me to my buried, fearful emotions of expecting to die or wanting to die—all related to the events of 9/11. As I discussed in Part One, while I didn't initially think that these were impacting me, and I had not been outwardly reactive, I did feel on many levels as though the events of 9/11 took away my sense of security. I also began to realize that part of me expected or wanted to die. As I reflected on this event, another aspect of the issue became clear to me. After 9/11, I spent long hours at my desk, surrounded by televisions that were endlessly replaying footage of the attack and delivering updates on the terrorist threat level. It's no wonder these emotions became deeply ingrained in my subconscious mind. After all, as you know from Step G, two of the main keys for reprogramming the subconscious mind are *repetition* and *emotional intensity*. The daily news was intense and repetitive. But it wasn't just the news; it was my pattern. Even after being injured, I was in so much pain and felt that I had no future, which further repeated my pattern of wanting to die.

As I continued to work with my mind and connect to my intuition, it became clear to me that expecting/wanting to die was the Symptom Emotion that my body had linked up to CRPS. This created feelings of fear in my nervous system. As you'll recall, in Chapter 6 I mentioned that it was like one part of my mind wanted to jump off a cliff while the other part knew it would be painful and deadly to do so.

Interestingly, the origin of CRPS can be traced back to the American Civil War, where it was first identified by Dr. Silas Weir Mitchell who found this medical condition in soldiers who had been wounded. Given their situation, I could see how it might be possible that their emotions may have been related to feelings of fear or an expectation of dying. There is no way to know for certain, of course.

While CRPS is not common, I have had a few people with CRPS attend my classes, workshops, and speaking engagements over the years, who also had similar emotional patterns of expecting or wanting to die. However, they too had no idea that these patterns were buried in their subconscious minds. Their emotions presented themselves in a variety of different ways; some were linked to trauma while others were not. For example, one woman's fiancé had died, and a part of her felt she wanted to die to be with him; yet another part of her felt a growing fear for her own mortality. In another case, a man carried extreme guilt, which created an underlying feeling that he did not deserve to live.

In some cases, a person's patterns toward dying can be found in their unconscious language patterns, such as saying in jest, "My [parent or spouse] is going to kill me," or "Don't kill me, but I made a mess in the kitchen." While this statement is typically not said with any seriousness (similar to the "joke" about being abandoned by a spouse in Chapter 6), the Symptom Emotion can have both "insignificant" light daily interactions as well as intense deeper emotions connected to the same patterned way of thinking and feeling.

The subconscious mind does not rationalize information; it simply acts on the *programming*. So if you repeat the phrase, "My mother is going to kill me" with emotional intensity, the feeling can start to become ingrained in your subconscious mind. This is not to say that your mother would actually harm you; rather, by repeating these words, your mind, body, and nervous system may internalize these emotions. And as a result, these emotions can attract more similar emotional energy to them. ("Like attracts like," as they say.) In my situation, I worked to dissolve any emotions that were connected to this patterned way of thinking and feeling because I no longer wanted to be drawn to (or attract) that similar emotional energy in my life anymore.

Since CRPS was my most pressing issue, I chose to tackle it first. By working with one issue at a time, it provided me with greater clarity. Then I proceeded to address my other ailments. I would recommend that you do the same and only work with one health issue at a time.

In addition to CRPS, I had several other low back issues, and the pain in my lower back had continued to worsen after my initial injury. As I was exploring the emotions connected to each ailment, I could also understand why my low back pain had worsened over the course of my illness. On a physical level, I was advised by my doctors that my back pain had increased due to weakness and muscle loss. True enough, but I also began to see the emotional connection. As you'll read in the coming pages, emotions relating to the back can relate to feelings of having a solid foundation in life. And I felt like my foundations in life continued to crumble the longer I was injured.

Logically Interpreting Back / Spine Issues

When I analyzed the spine using this same logical approach, I asked myself, *What does the spine, in general, do?* Anatomically, it supports our entire body and is like a pillar for our physical lives. Then, I thought more specifically about the function of the lower back, and I recognized that it supports and balances the weight of our bodies, thus our lives. I asked myself, *Do I feel stressed about feeling supported and balanced in life?*

As soon as I posed this question, the answer was clear. While I had wonderful people helping me, I also felt very unstable and unsupported. After all, I was injured, and no one could help me heal. Additionally, after the events of 9/11, I felt extremely unstable in life for a variety of reasons.

Throughout my years of working with people, I've continued to find that the emotions linked to low back pain often connect to feelings about being "supported." For instance, I've worked with people who felt unsupported by their spouses in their household or with their children. Others felt unsupported by their coworkers or family, or they experienced feelings of financial insecurity even if, in reality, they were financially secure. In some cases, people have negative emotions toward those who supported them, such as feeling guilty for getting angry or even feeling guilty about money. If you are experiencing low back pain, you could ask yourself if you have negative emotions about "support" in life.

For upper back pain, you could continue to think of the spine as a pillar and reflect on what you are placing on top of it. Are you feeling stressed or overwhelmed by the weight you are carrying? Do you feel burdened or angry about the responsibilities you have to bear?

If you still find it peculiar that different emotions can be connected to different parts of the back, it may be helpful to recall our discussion on p65, where we briefly discussed a study from 2022 that focused on police officers. In this study, the researchers observed that there were distinct emotions associated with upper back pain compared to lower back pain. In their study, they observed that police officers with low back pain felt unsupported, while officers with upper back pain experienced "stress."[5]

From this, we can see additional evidence that, even when it comes to back pain, different emotions can affect us in different ways. (If you wish to gain a deeper understanding on this topic, you can find a podcast episode on the book's website.)

Using this same logic, we can analyze scoliosis, which is a curvature of the spine. The common emotional link to this particular ailment has to do with feeling obligated or pressured to modify your life around something or someone else. I have worked with people who felt that they had to put their spouses, children, or parents first and were always forgoing their own desires.

Interestingly, our language patterns, including idioms, can also be useful to consider when you're identifying your Symptom Emotion. For example, a person might feel that they are "carrying a lot on their back" or that people are "on their back" if they feel someone is nagging them. As odd as it may sound, these emotions can impact your body and be subconsciously connected to your illness or injury, keeping your body from healing.

GIFT MIND-BODY HEALING CHART

To provide you with a deeper understanding of this mind-body emotional-energy connection, I have created a list of body parts, including a few emotional associations for each body part and some ideas of questions you could ask yourself (p198).

The aim of the chart is to provide you with a template so you can develop a new way of thinking about the mind-body emotional-energy connection, and then do what I did and logically interpret the message that your body is trying to tell you.

As you review the chart, you'll notice there are several body parts listed, and each body part has a range of several different interpretations. It is unlikely that you'll resonate with every interpretation that is listed under each body part. That's okay; you shouldn't expect to. This is akin to multiple people looking at a piece of art and each taking away different interpretations of it. The same is true here. You'll want to notice what comes up for you.

This chart is not meant to diagnose you or to be all-encompassing. Researchers estimate that there are over ten thousand different diseases and ailments, as well as thousands of body parts, so it simply wouldn't be possible—or practical—to list all of the associations and multiple interpretations here.[6] Furthermore, your goal here, at this stage, is not simply to get a list; it is also to master your mind and learn to think in a different way. This way you can feel empowered and build this skill which you can utilize for the rest of your life.

An Overview of the Mind-Body Emotional-Energy Connection Chart and Process:

- First, review the chart. I have provided you with a short list of body parts along with their corresponding general functions (e.g., the eyes are responsible for vision) and a set of sample "starter questions" designed to help guide your thinking process.
- Next, deepen your understanding. After the chart, I will provide you a few examples to assist you in doing so.
- Finally, identify your Symptom Emotion. I will guide you through a step-by-step process to help you logically interpret your own ailment, just as I did with mine.

In reviewing this template, you may find it eye-opening because you will start to see that there are common idioms all around us involving body parts. These can often be useful starting points which is why I've included them here. These idioms can help you begin to see your mind-body emotional-energy connection in a different way.

Learning to Think About Your Body in a New Way: Common Emotional Associations

ANKLES:

Basic Functions: To provide mobility, stability, and "up and down" movement of your feet.

Possible Emotional Associations: Emotions regarding your ability to move your life in the direction you want to go or stepping up in life.

Starter questions to ask yourself: Am I stressed about trying to elevate my life and/or walk in a new direction? Am I having difficulty lifting my life? Do I feel I am not allowed or am undeserving to step up or change direction in life? Am I trying to walk in a direction that is not wholly in integrity? Did I recently receive something that I feel undeserving of?

ARMS:

Basic Functions: Your arms help you move items as well as hug and hold people.

Possible Emotional Associations: Emotions regarding the people whom you wrap your arms around, such as children, spouse, and your community. Your ability and flexibility to move around/arrange your daily life the way you want it.

Starter questions to ask yourself: Do I have stress or guilt toward those whom I "hold in my arms" or "wrap my arms around?" Or guilt toward someone who I am keeping at "arm's length?" Do I have a tendency to push people away? Do I feel as though I do not have the ability to arrange my day the way I want it? Do I feel as though I have lost the ability to control my day-to-day life?

BACK / SPINE:

Basic Functions: Serves as the structure and pillar for our physical existence. Each part of the back can have a different emotional message. See below.

LOWER BACK:

Basic Functions: To support and stabilize the weight of your body.

Possible Emotional Associations: Emotions regarding things that support and add stability to the foundation of your life, such as your work, home, finances, and family.

Starter questions to ask yourself: Am I feeling unsupported at home or at work? Do I find myself getting mad at or feeling guilt toward those who are supporting me? Do I feel stress toward the things that are supporting me in life, such as job uncertainty? Do I feel financial worry or guilt for having too much money or too little or do I lack integrity with money? Do I feel unsupported, as though I have to do everything myself (even if it's not true)?

MIDDLE BACK:

Basic Functions: To set the structure for your body, stabilize your rib cage, and protect your organs.

Possible Emotional Associations: Emotions regarding structure and protection in life.

Starter questions to ask yourself: Do I feel it's hard to have structure or stability in my life? Do I feel that I need to "watch my back" or that people may "stab me in the back?" Do I feel that I have to protect myself from people doing things "behind my back?" Do I feel angry or a need to protect myself from people who are "on my back" about every little thing? Am I turning my back on others and feeling badly about it? Do I need to "grow a spine" because I feel I cannot speak up for myself or that it is painful to do so?

UPPER BACK:

Basic Functions: To help you stand up straight. (The top of the Pillar.)

Possible Emotional Associations: Emotions regarding your ability to stand tall, as well as what you feel is being placed upon you.

Starter questions to ask yourself: What or who do I feel like I am "carrying on my back?" Do I feel that it's bad to stand tall? Do I feel it's hard to stand tall because someone or something in life will just knock me down anyway? Do I feel confident that I can handle what I am carrying on my back? Do I feel upset because there is too much to handle, or because I am carrying too much on my back and it is painful or weighing me down? Am I carrying too much and it feels impossible to stand tall?

BOWEL:

Basic Functions: To absorb nutrients and fluids from what we take in, then expel the waste.

Possible Emotional Associations: Emotions regarding being able to absorb what you do need and let go of that which you no longer need.

Starter questions to ask yourself: Do I find it hard to let go of old issues? Do I find myself being unforgiving or holding longstanding grudges? If I am in a disagreement, do I dredge things up from the past to use against others? Am I stuck in the past in my relationships to such an extent that I still see people for who they used to be and not for who they are now? (For example, some people still see and treat their grown children as young kids.) Do I constantly remind myself of negative mistakes that others made in the past, thinking this will keep me safe and protected from them?

FACE:

Basic Functions: To enable you to express yourself and connect with others (through seeing, hearing, and speaking).

Possible Emotional Associations: Emotions regarding the way others see you and how you are seen.

Starter questions to ask yourself: Do I feel embarrassed, humiliated, or self-conscious? Do I feel hypercritical about the way the world sees me? Do I feel as though I have "lost face" (lost respect or feel humiliated), or that I "have egg on my face"? Is there someone I am not wanting to face?

FEET:

Basic Functions: To help us stand and absorb impact.

Possible Emotional Associations: Emotions regarding where you are standing in life and the impact of how you are being treated.

Starter questions to ask yourself: Am I tired of where I am standing in life? Do I feel that I have to defend my stance or stand up for myself against others? Do I feel that I am being treated unfairly or without respect, and that I just have to stand there and take it (absorb it)? Have I been feeling so upset that I want to put my "foot down" or stomp my feet? Or do I feel that I am "dragging my feet" or "digging in my heels" with resistance?

HANDS:

Basic Functions: To hold, grip, handle, or do specific tasks.

Possible Emotional Associations: Emotions regarding what you are holding, gripping, doing, or working on in life.

Starter questions to ask yourself: How do I feel about what I've "got my hands in," or what I am working on in life? Do I feel that others are critical of what I am doing or working on? Or the way I am doing it? Do I find myself trying to bend the rules in what I am doing? Am I feeling criticized or guilty for not doing enough or for not "giving people a hand" (helping them)? Do I feel frustrated and feel that my "hands are tied"? Am I gripping on to someone or something in an effort to control?

HEAD / BRAIN:

Basic Functions: To think and process information.

Possible Emotional Associations: Emotions regarding how you are thinking and processing information.

Starter questions to ask yourself: Do I tend to have "a lot on my mind" or "go over and over things in my head" so much that it hurts? Do I think in a way that is self-critical? Do I have negative thoughts that I am stewing on, such as thinking that everyone is against me or laughing at me or attacking me? Do I think about others in strategic or mean ways, such as wanting to manipulate or punish them? Do I feel that I am "beating my head against a wall," trying to achieve something without creating a more realistic approach? Do I find myself stuck in cyclical thinking, defending, arguing, justifying, or stewing about people or situations in life?

HEART:

Basic Functions: To pump blood (the river of life) and nutrients through your body.

Possible Emotional Associations: Emotions regarding the flow of both life and also the flow of love in life.

Starter questions to ask yourself: Do I feel that I want life to abruptly stop? Am I trying to stop the flow of love because someone I love died? Do I feel that the way life is flowing is too painful? Do I feel that I don't deserve that which is flowing into my life? Do I feel guilty for loving someone? Did I have a major trauma that disconnected me from the flow of life? Am I feeling imbalanced in the flow of life by wanting material objects and rejecting love and nurturing? Are my actions stopping the flow of love? Are material objects blocking the flow of love in my life?

HIPS:

Basic Functions: To provide stability where you are standing in life, to take large steps moving forward, and to be flexible in the way you move forward.

Possible Emotional Associations: Emotions regarding larger steps forward in life relating to the big picture.

Starter questions to ask yourself: Do I feel it is unsafe to make large steps moving forward? Or that there is not much life left to live? Do I stop myself from making changes because I feel apprehensive about my future? Do I feel there's nothing (or too little) to move forward to? Do I feel guilty or stressed about moving forward in life? Am I inflexible or rigid and set in my ways to the point that it causes issues within my relationships?

KNEES:

Basic Functions: The knees are required for most movements that we make as well as our ability to stand tall.

Possible Emotional Associations: Emotions regarding wanting to move forward and stand tall (to be proud and confident).

Starter questions to ask yourself: Am I trying to stand tall and proud while simultaneously feeling that I am not good enough or inferior? Am I criticizing, diminishing, or fault-finding in myself and/or others around me? Do I feel the need to protect or defend myself from criticism or attacks in order to stand tall? Do I have a pattern of attacking or reacting against those who are needed for my success (to stand tall)? Do I feel like someone has "brought me to my knees" (weakened or defeated) or "cut me off at the knees" (stopped in my efforts and/or my ability to succeed)?

LEGS:

Basic Functions: To enable you to stand and walk forward in life.

Possible Emotional Associations: Emotions regarding both where you are standing in life and how you are moving forward.

Starter questions to ask yourself: Do I feel that I can't "stand up for myself" in life? Do I feel that life is going to be hard moving forward and that there is a tough or painful road ahead? Do I feel afraid of moving forward or that there is no way to move forward in life?

LUNGS:

Basic Functions: To take in oxygen (life), pass the oxygen to your blood, and to exhale the old (carbon dioxide).

Possible Emotional Associations: Emotions regarding how you are taking in life and assimilating it.

Starter questions to ask yourself: Am I afraid of taking in life? Do I feel that things in life are happening so fast I cannot take them in easily or "catch my breath"? Do I feel that the rapid pace of events triggers feelings of urgency and uncertainty, leading to a sense of panic? Do I feel resentful because someone is rushing me? Does it feel like more than I can handle, and I "don't have a moment to breathe?" Do I feel that I am going to get in trouble for receiving good things in life? Is it more than I deserve to take in? Am I holding my breath in suspense, waiting for something to happen?

NECK:

Basic Functions: To provide flexibility to your skull so that you can scan your surroundings.

Possible Emotional Associations: Emotions regarding looking around in life; what direction you are looking toward or resisting and looking away from.

Starter questions to ask yourself: Am I resisting someone who I feel is a "pain in the neck" because they are nagging, needy, or _____? Am I resisting authority and turning my head away? Am I resisting people because of hurt feelings, overwhelm, frustration, business, or rebelliousness? Am I resisting someone because I feel they are too close and "breathing down my neck"?

SHOULDERS:

Basic Functions: To help you move your arms which enables you to perform tasks and carry objects in life.

Possible Emotional Associations: Emotions regarding everything you are doing in life and what you are responsible for carrying.

Starter questions to ask yourself: How do I feel about what I'm doing in life? Am I trying to do too many things at once? Do I feel pressure from everything I must do, as though I am "carrying the weight of the world on my shoulders?" Do I feel that I need to shoulder the responsibility for everything? Do I feel annoyed that someone is leaning or standing on my shoulders?

STOMACH:

Basic Functions: To take in food and begin breaking it down.

Possible Emotional Associations: Emotions regarding what you're having to swallow or digest in this moment.

Starter questions to ask yourself: Is there something in my life that I can't digest or "stomach"? Am I seeing things that disgust or bother me and make me feel "sick to my stomach"? Do I feel like things are being shoved down my throat and I just have to swallow them and say nothing? Do I have a "fire in my belly" (strong ambition or determination) to do something that is not good for me, such as attack another person? Do I feel so nervous about what I am taking in that I have "butterflies in my stomach"? Am I trying to consume something (or someone) that isn't rightfully mine? Do I have a habit of trying to take in too much at once?

UTERUS:

Basic Functions: Important for menstruation, fertility, and pregnancy.

Possible Emotional Associations: Feelings toward your romantic partner, children, or the idea of having children.

Starter questions to ask yourself: Am I reactive in my intimate relationships? Do I feel attacked or find myself attacking my partner? Do I notice myself being untruthful, misleading, or passive-aggressive in these relationships? Do I find that I am controlling or competitive in these relationships? Do I feel angry for not feeling supported and nurtured in these relationships and feel that no one is there for me?

WRIST:

Basic Functions: Provides range of motion and strength to your hands.

Possible Emotional Associations: Emotions regarding mobility, flexibility, ease, or strength/force that is needed to accomplish what you are doing or working on.

Starter questions to ask yourself: Do I feel like I have to apply a lot of force or effort to complete projects or get things done? Do I find myself trying to force others, twist circumstances, or possibly manipulate others to do or get what I want? Am I set in my ways or inflexible in what I am working on? Do I feel frustrated, as if other people are working against my efforts (so there is resistance from them), and they are stopping or hindering me from what I'm trying to accomplish?

LOGICALLY INTERPRETING YOUR PAIN OR DISEASE

Before we begin the process of identifying your Symptom Emotion, I want to share with you a few helpful examples of the "logical interpretation" approach. By doing so, you can start to get a broader picture of the power of the mind-body-emotional connection, as well as the function of your body and the emotional association.

Does Your Symptom Emotion Connect with an NPP?

Take a moment to recall Sofia, who had been trying to step into a new direction in life when she suffered from her ankle injury. As she and I began to explore what she was having a hard time stepping into, she mentioned she had made a mistake in the past. As a result, she felt guilty and undeserving of success. Sofia's NPP and her Symptom Emotion were directly connected; she felt guilty about the past (NPP) and therefore had a hard time stepping forward in a new direction in life (her Symptom Emotion).

Counterintuitive Circumstances Connected to Your Symptom Emotions

If we analyze broken heart syndrome (also known as takotsubo cardiomyopathy), it may initially seem straightforward to logically interpret it. After all, it's well-documented that a person can feel as though their heart is breaking from the loss of a loved one, which can result in triggering a heart-related illness.[7] Broken heart syndrome can also be connected to other traumatic events, such as a divorce, trauma, or car accident.

However, there are also rare cases in which a person can suffer the same type of heart issues except they're triggered by a positive event, such as a surprise or a wedding. You may wonder, *How is it possible for a positive event to impact someone in a negative way?* The reason is that a positive event could potentially be linked up to negative subconscious emotions. A person may feel undeserving, guilty, unsafe, or fearful of the particular positive circumstance, which could create feelings of wanting to stop the flow of life. And if you analyze the heart and think about its *function*, the heart's job is to pump blood and maintain the "flow of life." So, again we can see a possible logical connection.

As you dive into the logical approach, you'll want to keep in mind that while the body can extremely logical, the emotions themselves are not always logical.

Interpret the Ailment/Illness: A Logical Approach

Now it's your turn to interpret what valuable message your pain or illness is trying to communicate about what you'll need to change in order to heal yourself and your life.

In this process, you'll follow the same logical steps:

- Choose one pain, symptom, or illness that you're currently experiencing. You'll want to start with the most pressing challenge. Note which part of the body is affected by this.

- Then ask yourself, *What does this body part do? What is its function?*

- Now consider any emotions that could be associated with that function. (Refer to the chart starting on p198 to give you ideas for the interpreting process.) This might include asking yourself if there are any sayings or idioms about the body part in question that could give you clues as to the message your body is trying to give you.

- Next, ask yourself any pertinent questions related to the kind of emotional connections you find as per the style of the questions shown in the boxes.

For example, in the case of Aimee's shoulder injury, let's consider the function of the shoulders, which relates to what we do and what we feel responsible for carrying in life. Aimee could ask herself, "Is there something or someone for whom I feel responsible in life?" or "Is there someone or something that I feel burdened by and that I am carrying on my shoulders?" This would have led her to think about her husband, as she felt he was a burden.

Furthermore, Aimee could have made a logical connection with the rotator cuff tear itself. If she had analyzed the rotator cuff, which simply stated, connects the arm to the shoulder joint, she could have realized that the arms symbolize the people we hold close. This realization would also have led her to her husband, as she had figuratively held him close for years. However, now she wanted to "tear" away from him because he was a burden. Through this perspective, we can observe the logic behind her Symptom Emotion. From this, she was clear on her Symptom Emotion and went on to use the rest of the steps in the GIFT Method to release and transform herself.

- If you have identified the Symptom Emotion for your ailment or injury at this stage, fantastic! Write down your findings and make sure that you don't slide into any of the negative emotions right now. It can be useful to do the

Stress Interrupt and Freedom Technique (SIFT; p175) to lessen the intensity of your Symptom Emotion and allow you to move forward easily. Feel free to skip ahead to the exercise titled "Introducing Your 180° Shift." (p217)

- If you haven't yet received any obvious insights or answers to identify your Symptom Emotion, please don't worry. There are additional resources that may be more aligned with the way your mind works, such as the intuitive approach that follows.

AN INTUITIVE APPROACH TO EXPLORE YOUR SYMPTOM EMOTION

Prior to my injury, I'd held the false belief that intuition was simply a gut feeling, and since I knew that feelings were not always accurate, by deductive reasoning, it seemed silly or even dangerous for me to operate my life based on a gut feeling. However, after this process of self-healing unfolded, I began to understand intuition in a new way—as I mentioned previously, I began to see it as a skill that we all have and are born with. Much like children grow up and stop using their imagination (having imaginary tea parties), we start ignoring our intuition because we don't realize we have it. So, if you have disconnected from your intuition as most people have, you will want to remember to be patient with yourself and have an open mind.

Everyone's mind works differently; therefore one person may receive intuitive messages in a different way from another. Some of us tend to be more visual, some more sound-focused (auditory), while others of us are more feeling-focused (kinesthetic), and so on.

Intuitive information about your Symptom Emotion may come from the dominant intuitive "language" that your mind prefers. For example, a visual person may be more likely to receive intuitive messages via images or visions. Other times, messages may come in a mix of the various "languages" For example, you may "hear" an answer and also receive a vision. The important thing to keep in mind for the "Ask the Ailment" exercise (below) is to be open to any and all messages of intuition that you encounter, in whatever form they may take, or however faint or subtle they may feel.

Ask the Ailment:
An Intuitive Approach

To be successful in working with your intuitive abilities, you must have a calm mind. For this reason, I suggest that as you go through this exercise, take your time with it, and make it a point to be patient, kind, and loving toward yourself.

- First, find a quiet place where you won't be disturbed. Take a few deep breaths to relax and settle into the present moment. Then focus your thoughts on your breathing and your heartbeat.

- Rub your fingers together or squeeze your toes together, noticing how it feels to be grounded in your body.

- Tune in to the area of your body where the pain or ailment you want to focus on is located, then "ask" your ailment if there is something it would like to "tell" you. I would not suggest asking this question aloud because the contrast of the spoken word may feel loud in a quiet place. It may also make your brain feel as though you are listening for a normal-sounding auditory voice, which, in most cases, you will not receive. Instead, you can suggest this question to your body by thought, *Is there something you are trying to tell me or that I need to know?*

- Next, relax and pay attention to anything that comes to mind in answer to this question, no matter how subtle—via physical sensations, visions, memories, emotions, songs, or whatever else.

- If you receive any information or guidance, great. You'll want to jot it down so that you can take time to analyze and understand the specific meaning as well as any *emotions* that arise from it.

To illustrate how to do this, I will share with you an example from Jada, a woman who suffered from fibroids.

When Jada did this exercise and asked her body for the message, she had a vision of arguing with her partner. She immediately recognized this as a pattern in her relationship, but she hadn't realized it could be affecting her physical health. However, once she received this intuitive vision, she began to examine her emotions around her relationship more closely and wondered if they could indeed be the issue.

Jada cross-referred this intuitive approach with the "logical interpretation" approach from earlier and was able to uncover how the affected body part was connected to the issue. She had uterine fibroids; therefore, upon reflection on the uterus and its functions, she could see the connection. She thought about how the function of the uterus, which is for pregnancy and childbirth, as well as preparing itself each month to receive an embryo. Therefore it made sense to analyze her emotions regarding her relationships with her children and/or a romantic partner. She also thought about a fibroid, which is a mass of cells that are growing and dividing. Jada put the two together and saw that she had a massive amount of hurt and anger she was harboring deep inside, and it was proliferating and boiling over. Jada felt confident that this was her Symptom Emotion and began to work through the rest of the GIFT Method to begin genuinely releasing and transforming this growing anger that was festering.

If any Symptom Emotion insights come up for you during this process, you'll want to make sure to write them down so that you have the information saved and also to avoid going into any of the negative emotions at this moment. If something comes up for you that you're not quite sure about, or if you had multiple possibilities come up, then you can double-check it with the logically "Interpret the Ailment" approach from earlier (p208) and see which emotion makes logical sense. Or you can use some of the additional tools that follow.

- If you haven't found any Symptom Emotion insights or answers yet, don't worry. Some people will get an answer using the intuitive approach, while others won't. Similar to learning how to ride a bicycle, it can take practice to develop this skill which you can continue to work on if you'd like. For now, you can use another tool to help you identify your Symptom Emotion.

Note: if you find that you are being impatient with yourself, it would be best to take a break and use the SIFT Technique and then also embrace the willingness to change. I want to emphasize this because as you may already know, impatience is a growing issue in our world. In fact, if you do a quick internet search and type in "society of instant gratification," you will find one article after another on this topic. Unfortunately, impatience has become a programmed way of thinking for many people. If you approach your intuition from this mindset, you will likely not get the answers you are seeking. Part of the problem with this expectation of instant gratification is that many people can get frustrated or agitated if they don't have the answer instantly. And these can be the very feelings that block you. I personally did not know the answers when I was healing myself. I just kept clearing my mind and following through. I let go of my impatience and turned it into pure determination to uplift myself as much as I could. As I did, I was able to gain more clarity to see the answers that were needed to heal myself. If I had been impatient, I likely would have failed. So please remember that it's important to be patient and kind to yourself.

Note: Another common reason for impatience is intermittent follow through. In this case a person might follow through for periods of time, but not consistently. The problem is that if you are not working on embracing change each and every day, it's hard to succeed because your progress doesn't typically "pause." Instead you will likely slip back into your old patterns.

This would be akin to setting out on a road trip from New York to California, and somewhere along the way you decide to take a break. During your break your subconscious mind sends you back toward New York (because that is your norm). Now you're driving in the wrong direction without realizing it. Then you decide to start driving to California again and have to almost start over. As you can imagine, if a person was really wanting to arrive in California, this could be a frustrating road trip.

With this in mind, at any point during the process, if you notice that you keep going back into your old patterns, you will want to remind yourself to stay consistent with your mind reprogramming. As you do, it can feel exciting instead of frustrating. Continuing with the analogy, if you stay consistent, you will start to notice road signs signaling that you are getting closer to California. Or, in the case of your health, you may see signs such as improved blood tests, decreased pain, more energy, and less fatigue, etc. Use these signs as an opportunity to celebrate yourself. With each progression forward, it becomes easier to stay out of impatience and instead have a growing sense of excitement to continue to follow through.

Additional Resources to Expand Your Mind

There are a few additional tools and resources that you can use to further develop your connection with your body and your energy or to help you identify your Symptom Emotion if you have not done so yet.

Bonus Short Video Course

If you go online to BrandyGillmore.com/SpecialAccess, you'll be able to find a short but powerful video course that will teach you another way to ask questions of, and get answers from, your body and connect further with the energy of your body.

Podcast Episodes

I wanted people around the world to be able to witness this incredible ability that we have to transform our own health and life, so I started a podcast. On it, I work with live volunteers and show them how to use their own minds to release their pain and ailments on the spot!

Many people have found this to be a valuable resource for their own understanding and clarity around using the GIFT Method. As people hear the stories of others and witness their transformative experiences, it often leads to further insights and breakthroughs into their own awareness, healing, and transformation. For this reason, I strongly recommend either listening to a podcast episode or watching a video showing thermal imaging, so you can observe the process and gain additional insights yourself. When you listen to the podcast, keep in mind that when I check into my own intuition, the word "bingo" comes through. Therefore, you're likely to hear me say the word with some frequency while I am coaching people to heal themselves with their minds.

Continue to Unblock Your Mind

If you have not yet identified your Symptom Emotion, then likely your mind may be blocked. It never feels good to be emotionally blocked, but the good news is that if you don't dwell on it, you can work to unblock your mind. This is crucial progress toward your healing. If you are feeling blocked, it would be best to proceed with the rest of the GIFT Method in the pages that follow, with a direct focus on releasing the emotions that can block you. The two most common blocks that I have found are feelings of fear and NPP. Therefore, if you identified any NPP in Chapter 10 or have underlying feelings of fear, I strongly recommend prioritizing these issues. This can help you unblock your mind and make progress with your healing.

Note: After you work to free yourself from your NPP and/or feelings of fear, and your mind feels less blocked, come back to the "Interpret the Ailment" and/or "Ask the Ailment" exercises to see if you can more clearly identify your Symptom Emotion. Then, once you identify your specific Symptom Emotion, you'll want to follow through to apply the upcoming exercises to your Symptom Emotion so you can begin to transform it.

INTRODUCING YOUR 180° SHIFT: THE IMPORTANCE OF CREATING POSITIVE SHIFTS AS SOON AS POSSIBLE

Once you've identified a Symptom Emotion and reduced the intensity of it with the SIFT Technique if required, remember not to "hang out" in the negativity. This is also true if you are working with a different emotion, such as your NPP. Instead, you'll want to immediately identify how you *want* to feel. While this is simple and logical, it is also profound. Most people identify the negative and immediately want to work to release it, but they never get clear on how they want to feel instead. In most cases, this keeps them stuck because they cannot reprogram their mind to think and feel in a new way. But if you consciously decide on how you want your mind to think and feel and then reprogram your mind to do that, you will set yourself up for success and make it much easier for your mind to let the old pattern go completely.

For this reason, before you jump into the steps of freeing yourself from the negative, you will want to identify the new, positive way that you want to feel.

This is what I refer to as your 180° Shift.

As the name implies, this involves identifying the new emotional "shift" that would move you in the opposite direction from your Symptom Emotion.

For example, if you identified feeling fearful as something you want to free yourself from, then you'll want to choose feelings of safety as your 180° Shift.

It's important to note here that some emotions don't have an exact opposite. In that case, you'll just want to choose a contrasting emotion that feels most relevant to your Symptom Emotion. For example, if your Symptom Emotion is anger, you could choose feelings of kindness, calm and understanding for your new 180° Shift.

The relevancy of the 180° Shift that you choose will be key. After all, imagine if Sofia—the woman who didn't feel deserving to step into her success—had selected Eli's 180° Shift of feeling supported. While this would have been positive mind programming, it wouldn't have worked to help her heal as it wouldn't have been relevant or specific enough to address her underlying Symptom Emotion, and therefore her specific ailment of ankle pain.

Some examples of relevant and specific 180° Shifts are:

- Aimee felt unloved, so her 180° Shift was to bring in a feeling that she was very loved.
- Eli felt unsupported in life and also financially insecure, so his 180° Shift was to bring in feelings that he was supported as well as feelings of financial safety.
- Sofia felt undeserving, so her 180° Shift was to bring in the feelings of deserving success and being free to enjoy that success.
- Jada felt hurt, angry, and reactive with her spouse, so her 180° Shift was feeling that her relationship was harmonious, kind, and loving, and that she and her partner were working together as a team.

Identify Your 180° Shift

It's now your turn to identify what a relevant 180° Shift would be for your Symptom Emotion, NPP, or any other underlying negative emotion so that you can begin to transform the problem into a gift. To do so, you can simply:

- Think about the specific Symptom Emotion, NPP, or other negative emotion that you've identified.

- Next, feel into what the best 180° Shift would be for the emotion that you're focusing on.

- In order to start getting your new 180° Shift programmed into your mind, you will want to integrate it into your uplifting Step G Techniques that you've been working with so far.
  - o First, review your current Power Vision (p118) and see if it already includes this feeling you've targeted for your 180° Shift. (Aimee's initial vision already included feeling loved, which was her 180° Shift.) If it does, great. If it does not already include this new positive emotion, then you can either add this feeling into your existing Power Vision or create a *new* Power Vision that includes this new 180° Shift feeling.
  - o Next, make your 180° Shift emotion one of your new Positive Emotional Patterns (p119).
  - o Use the Visual Reality Technique (p136) and choose a song with the NT Music Technique (p144).
  - o If you would like, you can also use Power Writing (p173) to help reinforce the new feeling.

As you are working on integrating your 180° Shift into your life, if you notice that your daily actions and behaviors are fueling your unwanted negative Symptom Emotion, then you'll want to discontinue this behavior to the best of your ability. For example:

- If your Symptom Emotion is a pattern of anger, then it would be best to avoid going into this emotional state as much as you can. If you know of a situation that frequently triggers you, then you'll want to clarify ahead of time how you'll respond differently. This way, you can do your best to try to avoid the trigger until you can fully release it.
- If your NPP includes actions such as taking your frustrations out on others or engaging in passive-aggressive behavior (see p164 for a list of examples of NPP), then you'll want to abstain from this behavior as much as possible while you work to fully reprogram your mind for lasting change in the coming steps.

In order to turn the positive feeling into a lasting positive pattern, I suggest using the combination of exercises you have chosen for at least thirty days or until you have healed yourself, whichever is longer.

Summary of the Key Exercises in This Chapter

- Identify your Symptom Emotion by using the "Interpret the Ailment" and/or the "Ask the Ailment" exercises. Remember to be kind and loving to yourself.
- If you haven't yet identified your Symptom Emotion, be patient with yourself. Continue with the rest of the techniques and work to unblock your mind by freeing yourself from NPP and fear.
- If you want additional help, refer to my online video guidance and podcast content to help you identify your Symptom Emotion.
- Make sure that you have identified a 180° Shift for each negative emotion you are working on. (This includes your Symptom Emotion, NPP, or fear.) Then follow through to begin reprogramming these changes.

STEP F OF THE GIFT METHOD: FREE YOURSELF

In this step we will focus on:

- Using the Emotional Brushing Technique to begin freeing yourself from negative emotional energy
- Learning your MBSS Needs
- Understanding and freeing yourself from miswired mind programming
- Factor 4 of the 5 Factors for GIFT Mind-Body Healing

This step includes:

Chapter 12
Free Yourself From Negative Emotional Energy

Chapter 13
Free Yourself from "Miswired"
Mind Programming

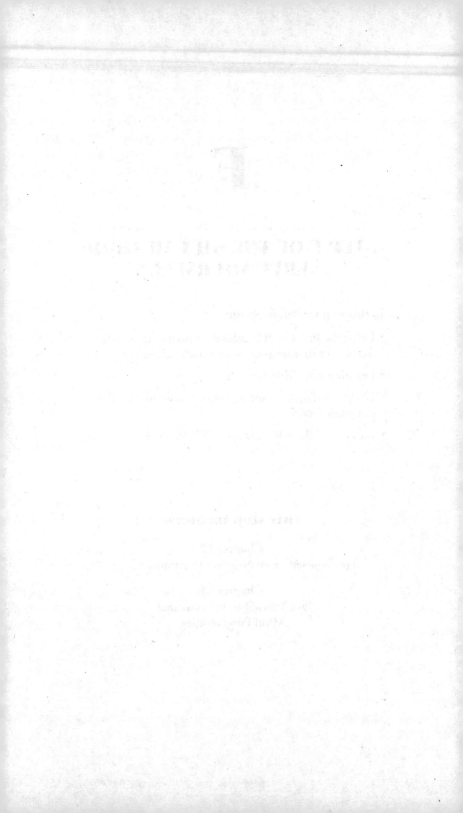

STEP F

12

FREE YOURSELF
FROM NEGATIVE
EMOTIONAL ENERGY

*The great decisions of human life have as a rule far more to do
with the instincts and other mysterious unconscious factors
than with conscious will and well-meaning reasonableness.*

—Carl Jung[1]

By this point, you'll want to have identified at least one unwanted
negative emotion that is stressing your body, blocking your
mind, or preventing you from healing yourself. Now, as we go
through this step, you'll want to begin freeing yourself from it.

To do so, it's important to start with the awareness that
these negative emotions can be part of a cycle (the Emotion-
Perception Cycle as discussed on p97). As you'll recall, in short,
negative emotions get stored in our subconscious minds and the
pattern repeats in our lives. In this case, we can store up even

more negative emotions and "stress" which can then render our minds unable to see the problem with the level of clarity that we need to change it. For this reason, to begin freeing yourself from the problem, it's important to first work on *decreasing* the unwanted negative emotions that have been clandestinely shaping your perception. The more you can free yourself and your mind from the influence that these negative emotional patterns have over you, the more you can gain the mental clarity that is needed in order to make a real change.

BREAKING FREE FROM THE EMOTION-PERCEPTION CYCLE

A simple way to illustrate the benefits of freeing your mind in this way is to first observe what occurs when a person is experiencing intense negative emotions. Imagine the following scenario: Your partner or spouse comes home angry about an argument they've just had with their mother. Your partner is so upset that they begin venting all their frustrations. As they're venting, in the middle of their upset, you start giving them advice. In that exact moment, how well do you think they would receive your advice? In most cases, not well—which you may have experienced if you've ever tried to do this.

Why does this happen? When a person is triggered, upset, or in a strong negative emotional state, their mind is typically not resourceful or open to new perspectives. Moreover, attempting to offer advice to them could potentially exacerbate their emotional response, leading to increased agitation, defensiveness, or even anger toward you.

However, continuing with this example, once your partner calms down, they may be more rational and open to new ideas or even think of some solutions themselves because their brain is in a more resourceful state. This simple scenario exemplifies the profound awareness that negative emotions can block our mind's ability to be resourceful and find solutions.

If we expand on this awareness and apply it to our emotional patterns, we can begin to understand what is happening at a deeper level of our minds and the reasons we can get stuck in the Emotion-Perception Cycle.

Similar to this scenario, long-standing patterns can keep our minds unresourceful and stuck in the same patterned way of thinking, feeling, and believing, even if we are not consciously aware of it. This can shape our beliefs about our world, ourselves, and others, as well as influence our actions which further keeps us locked into the pattern.

Most people will not recognize they are stuck in a pattern and will continue to reinforce negative beliefs, such as, "That's how life is," or "That's just how people are," or "That's just how my mom is." As we've discussed, these patterns can be hard to discern because many began in childhood.

Using Aimee's example with her husband, it was only after she began to *decrease* the negative emotions she felt toward her husband (by using the Freedom Techniques), that she was able to see with more clarity that the pattern had started in her childhood with her father. This clarity enabled her to use the rest of the steps of the GIFT Method to reprogram the entire pattern in her subconscious mind in order to make a real shift in her health and her life.

That is the importance of this chapter and of the Freedom Techniques. As you use these techniques, you can begin to decrease the hold that your negative patterns have over you so that you can access a more resourceful perspective to begin seeing and feeling in an entirely different way. True freedom awaits.

The Stress Interrupt and Freedom Technique (SIFT)

Freedom Technique 1

You've already been introduced to the first Freedom Technique on p175 of Chapter 10, where the Stress Interrupt and Freedom Technique (SIFT) was recommended as a way to immediately start addressing and letting go of any NPP that you may have identified at that stage.

Now, in this step, you can use the SIFT Technique on your Symptom Emotion, or you can use it to decrease *any* of the other negative emotions in your daily life. The more you can stay out of the negative and instead remain feeling uplifted and optimistic throughout your day, the more this can become your new norm. This, in turn, can help you get your body into its optimal state for self-healing.

The Emotional Brushing Technique

Freedom Technique 2

This powerful exercise can help you decrease/release your negative emotions, so that you can begin to shift the emotions affecting your health and life. As the name suggests, this technique involves using a physical "brushing" motion. This can help you feel the emotional shift in your mind, as well as in your body and nervous system.

- To begin with, identify one specific negative emotion or situation that you want to work on. It could be your NPP, Symptom Emotion, or any other negative emotion that you feel may be affecting you or that you are currently experiencing in your daily life.

- Bring your awareness to the negative emotion (how it feels in your body).

- Then place your hand against the middle of your breastbone and brush it downward, from your breastbone to your waist, keeping your hand firmly against your body. Imagine brushing off dust from your body. If you'd like a visual instruction for this technique, you can go to Brandygillmore. com/bookbonuses.

  Do this between five and ten times—or until the feeling of the negative emotion starts to reduce. As you're brushing down, you'll want to keep your awareness focused on how the negative emotion *feels* in your body (as opposed to being in your head or focusing on the event that took place). Continue brushing down while allowing the emotion to dissipate as much as possible.

- Next, perform the same firm downward brushing action five to ten times on the *left* side of your torso, moving from your underarm to your waist, until the feeling of the negative emotion subsides further.

- Next, do the same firm brushing-down action five to ten times on the *right* side of your torso, again moving from your underarm to your waist until the feeling of the negative emotion subsides further.

- If you are working on your Symptom Emotion, you may also want to brush down five to ten times over the specific area of any injury or ailment (if you have one)—until the feeling of the negative emotion you've been focusing on starts to dissipate further. For example, if your knee is injured, you could also brush down on your knee.

- Once you've brushed down at all three or four locations, repeat the action in all locations for a second time. But this time, actively remind your brain each time as you brush down that the negative feeling you're focusing on is not serving you, and that you're ready to let it go. To do this, you can repeatedly say something like: "*I see that this* _____ *[insert relevant negative emotion] is not serving me in any way. It's not going to help me now or in the future. I never need it again. It is not keeping me safe or helping me. I'm willing to let go of it completely.*"

- Next, change your statement to past tense and create a shift. To do this, you'll want to continue brushing down, alternating between the same locations on the body, and say, "*I used to feel_____ [insert the same negative emotion], but I now see that no longer makes sense. I let that feeling go. I now feel* _____ *[insert your 180° Shift (the new relevant desired positive emotion)].*"

Note: If you want to release your negative emotions toward a particular event or memory that is stuck in your mind, then you'll want to use the Emotional Brushing Technique toward *any* and *all* of the emotions that are connected to that memory.

For example, let's say you were yelled at by your boss, which generated several negative emotions. To begin shifting out of this heaviness, you'd want to remember that your emotions influence your thoughts. Instead of focusing on the circumstances that took place, you'd want to calm and free yourself from negative emotions. To do so, start using the Emotional Brushing Technique as we did previously (brushing down in each location on the body).

After you've used the Emotional Brushing Technique to address your feelings about the event in general, you'll want to notice if there are any other people or objects in that same memory that may have also triggered emotions. If so, brush down toward them too. For example, if there was a coworker standing nearby which resulted in feelings of embarrassment, then you'd want to brush down on your feelings toward the coworker as well as anything else, releasing any and all emotional charge that is connected to that memory.

Note: If you would like an additional Freedom Technique to help you release stubborn negative emotions, I have provided one for you on my website.

You may be wondering, do I need another release technique? The answer is that it depends on you. The reason it can be helpful is because our minds can store information in a variety of ways. For example, a person may smell a scent, such as apple pie, and experience a surge of emotions about their grandmother who used to bake apple pie. Extremely intense emotions can store up in your mind in a different way as well. If you'd like, you can access an advanced technique at: brandygillmore.com/advanced-release.

- After you implement the Freedom Techniques, the final step will be to bring your focus back to your positive mind programming by following through with your Step G Techniques. If you were working on releasing your Symptom Emotion, then it would be best to also make a point of reinforcing your new 180° Shift.

The See Mind Technique

After successfully reducing negative emotions, which is crucial for breaking free from the Emotion-Perception Cycle, it's time to implement the See Mind Technique. This powerful technique enables you to shift your mind away from what you no longer want and instead helps program it toward that which you do want. To implement it, simply:

- Decide on a specific new positive emotion that you want to start shifting your mind toward. (You'll want to choose one of your Positive Emotional Patterns from your Step G Techniques or your 180° Shift.)

- Next, make a point of consciously looking for evidence that can help you reinforce the positive emotion. For example, let's say your Symptom Emotion is fear. After using the Freedom Techniques, you'd use this technique to reinforce your 180° Shift, which, presumably, would be feeling safe. To implement this exercise, you'd point out evidence to your mind that our world is safe. Then, you'd intentionally embrace both the awareness and emotions as much as possible. Remember, the more you shift your emotions, the more you can shift your perception.

You can use this technique to reinforce any positive shift you are wanting to make. If you have felt that love is not safe, or that people are not nice, then purposely find and point out evidence to your mind that love is safe or that people are nice to begin shifting your emotions and perception.

You might be able to find real-life examples in your current environment. If not, you'll want to do your best to think of real-life examples and bring them to mind. Whether you find them readily available or need to consciously seek them out, the more you keep the examples grounded and realistic, the better.

Since your mind has been accustomed to focusing on the opposite (the negative), it may (or may not) feel hard to see the positive at first. If it is, think of it like a word search puzzle. The more you do it, the better your mind will get at it. Similarly, the more you intentionally seek out evidence of your 180° Shift, the better your mind will get at it. Of course, unlike a word search puzzle, in this case, your goal will be to program in the associated emotions as intensely as you possibly can so you can train your brain to begin seeing and feeling in a new way.

- With each piece of evidence you're able to find, you'll want to point it out to your mind and then really feel it as much as you can. Using this example, you would say, "*See, mind, it is safe.*" Then, feel it. You can insert any emotion: "*See, mind, it is* _____ *[insert new feeling]*." I understand this may sound extremely simple, but that's the point. When using these techniques, you will not want to overthink it. Instead, your goal is to place your focus on the emotions and the image. The more you can think about real-life experiences, feel them strongly, and get them in your mind with repetition, the easier it will be to create a pivotal shift. When this occurs, you will want to make a point to see the reference/evidence that you are giving to your mind while simultaneously allowing yourself to fully feel those feelings as much as you can, repeatedly, to program the new emotions into your mind.

To share an example of this technique, I'll introduce you to a man named Anthony who was in one of my classes. He had been diagnosed with ME/CFS (chronic fatigue syndrome).

His condition was so debilitating that he had been bedridden or confined to the couch for nearly seven years. It turned out that subconsciously, he was afraid of people. He felt they were cold-hearted and unkind, and he expected them to be cruel to him. Unbeknownst to him, these subconscious thoughts and emotions were shaping his perception of the world and impacting his health.

Once he gained awareness of his fearful perspective of the world during Step I, he knew he had to shift it in order to heal. He began to implement the See Mind Technique every day to begin programming feelings of safety into his mind.

To do this, he brought to mind images of people outside walking their dogs, couples in love, kids playing in parks and riding their bikes, families connecting, people helping others, and so on. As he thought about each of these safe, positive, and loving scenarios, he purposely noted to his mind, "*See, mind, it's safe.*" Then he focused on taking in the corresponding feelings and feeling them as strongly as possible.

The more he followed through with this exercise (as well as the other exercises), the more it began to shift his mindset of fear and worry to one of safety in life.

While these good things had always been there, his mind hadn't been able to notice them because he had been stuck for so long in an Emotion-Perception Cycle of fear and gloom. As he followed through consistently each day and also continued to shift his Symptom Emotion, he noticed a remarkable improvement in his health. His daily energy levels increased exponentially. To maintain lasting results and take his health to the next level, he needed to reprogram his mind at an even deeper level, which we'll be working on in the next chapter.

Summary of the Key Exercises in This Chapter

- To help reduce/release the intensity of your negative emotions, use the Freedom Techniques (Stress Interrupt and Freedom Technique and the Emotional Brushing Technique) at least three times a day or more often if feeling stressed. Apply them to your NPP, Symptom Emotion, or any other negative emotion you are currently experiencing.
- Use the See Mind Technique at least two times per day, every day, for at least thirty days. As you do, be sure to amplify your emotional energy in order to begin creating a radical shift in your emotions and perception.
- Continue with your Step G Techniques.

STEP F

13

FREE YOURSELF FROM "MISWIRED" MIND PROGRAMMING

The hunger for love is much more difficult to remove than the hunger for bread.

—*Mother Teresa*[1]

Now that you've started using the Freedom Techniques to decrease and release your negative emotions, your goal in this chapter will be to reprogram these unwanted emotional patterns in your subconscious mind so that you can free yourself from them once and for all. To do that, it is important for you to understand your Mind-Body-Soul-Spirit Emotional-Energy Needs (or MBSS Needs) because they can unconsciously influence every part of your life.

You may wonder how it is possible for the MBSS Needs to influence every aspect of our lives. The reason is because the

MBSS Needs are emotions we innately require, such as love and safety. On a positive note, if these emotions are programmed correctly, they can promote healing. However, issues arise when these emotions become miswired. For example: if the mind is programmed that it is unsafe to love or that negative emotions provide protection (e.g., holding onto hurt, fear, or trauma to stay safe). In this case, negative emotions can become impossible to release, and they can keep us from meeting our emotional-energy needs in healthy ways.

YOUR BODY'S EMOTIONAL ENERGY NEEDS

It may sound odd that our bodies physically *need* certain emotions. However, based on research, we can see evidence that specific emotions, such as love, are needed for optimal health. In fact, research has shown that a lack of love and human connection can lead to increased illness and even premature death in infants and in people of all ages.[2-6]

It is also well-known that if we lack feelings of safety (feeling unsafe/stressed), this can trigger the release of stress hormones. This is just one way these emotions can negatively impact the health of the body. During my injury, as I was researching feelings of fear, I was surprised to find that the phrase "scared to death" was more than just a saying. Indeed, a person can, in extreme cases, be so scared that their body releases fatal amounts of stress chemicals, causing death.[7]

Although this example may seem extreme, it highlights the importance of specific emotions, such as safety, which are vital. Think of the MBSS Needs as being like "emotional-energy food" for our bodies. Plants demonstrate the need for "energetic food" beautifully. They rely on water, essential nutrients from the soil, and also light energy from the sun for photosynthesis. Without this sufficient "energetic food," a plant will wither away and die.

Our human needs are similar. We need food, water, and sun, and we also have energetic and emotional needs that support our health. As we discussed, feelings of love and safety are two (out of four) of the emotional-energy needs to consider. As we discussed in Chapter 5, certain positive emotions can even trigger the release of biochemicals that are essential for optimal health. Therefore, it is crucial to ensure that you have these positive emotions (as well as your other MBSS Needs) programmed into your subconscious mind in positive ways.

It's no wonder that human beings will do whatever it takes to acquire feelings of love and safety—because we physically need them. And much like a plant will grow in the direction of the sun, humans will do whatever it takes to grow in the direction of these needs, even if it does not make logical sense. For this reason, these MBSS Needs unconsciously influence our actions, emotions, health—and, ultimately, our lives.

AN IMPORTANT INSIGHT FOR RELEASING UNWANTED NEGATIVE PATTERNS

The importance of this step is twofold. The first goal is to make sure that you are fulfilling these emotional-energy needs in positive ways that promote health and healing. The second goal is to ensure that you reprogram any unhealthy mind programming that is holding on to negative emotions or illness. This is what I refer to as "errored" or "miswired" mind programming.

While it may sound odd that our minds can become miswired, this is very common. For example, a person may have a traumatic experience, such as a car accident, and their mind may feel that it will keep them safe to hold on to the traumatic feelings in order to stay on high-alert and avoid the problem in the future. Others may have gotten their feelings hurt in a relationship and, as a result, their mind will hold on to the hurt to keep them "safe" so they don't get into another relationship.

We can also observe this unfortunate problem with traumatic situations, such as child abuse. The subconscious mind may get programmed to hold on to the wounding in order to remember to protect themselves from people in an effort to stay safe. However, holding on to these negative emotions can result in the opposite of safety; they can be detrimental to a person's well-being. Sadly, research shows that child abuse can increase a person's chances of suffering from both physical and mental illness.[8] Further, if we consider the awareness that buried emotions can repeat in our lives, it is clear that holding on to the abuse (or any trauma) will not keep a person safe. Referring back to the statistics on abuse from Chapter 6 (p77), you may recall that as many as 77 percent of people who experience abuse as an adult have also been abused during their childhood.

You might think that our minds would not become programmed to do something to our own detriment, right? However, that is not the case. It's important to remember that our subconscious minds do *not* store information based on logic. We previously discussed the example of a person who engages in self-harm. This is typically as a result of a past traumatic experience. In this case, a person can cut themselves and experience a variety of different *positive* emotions, such as relief, safety, and control.[9]

Of course, the person did not want to program this miswired information into their mind. Yet once the miswiring has occurred, it can influence their emotions and actions.

Based on the examples we've discussed so far, you may be thinking that miswired mind programming only pertains to safety; however, you may (or may not) be surprised to know that we can choose love over safety.

We can also observe this common behavior among children. Imagine a young boy who is with a group of friends. They challenge him to engage in a dangerous activity, and the boy stops because he is afraid for his safety. However, his group of friends call him a "chicken." What typically happens? With enough peer pressure, the boy will follow through with the dangerous act, ultimately placing his connection to others and his emotional safety *above* his physical safety. As we can see, these subconscious Needs control our emotions, actions, and behaviors.

There are other ways that miswired mind programming can affect you as well. For example, knowing that we need both love and safety, consider what happens if a person is programmed to feel that it's not safe to be hugged or to receive love. Or what if a person is hugging someone but deep down this also triggers their Symptom Emotion, such as feelings of resentment? Resolving miswired mind programming and meeting your MBSS Needs in healthy ways will be crucial for your success in getting your body to heal itself.

The problem is that if our minds are programmed to feel that negative emotions are keeping us safe (or meeting any of our other MBSS Needs), then no matter how hard we try to release them, our subconscious mind will hold on to them until we reprogram our minds that it is safer to let them go.

REPROGRAMMING YOUR AUTOMATIC EMOTIONAL REFLEXES

Another reason that these subconscious patterns can be difficult to resolve is because they are automatic. The easiest way to think about your *automatic* emotional programming is to first think about our automatic *physical* programming. For example, if a ball is thrown and it's coming toward your face, what would you do?

You would *physically* react!

You may immediately dodge it or catch it before you even have a chance to think and register what's happening. Why? Because we *need* to feel safe, and conveniently, you already have the feeling programmed into your subconscious mind that getting hit in the face with a ball is not safe. So, in this case, your subconscious programming comes to your rescue. This is an example of positive mind programming. In contrast, a young child who does not yet have this information programmed into their mind and nervous system would not respond in the same way. This simple example demonstrates that we have physical reflexes programmed into our minds to help keep us safe.

Similarly, we have what I refer to as "emotional reflexes," which are emotions that we automatically experience before we have a chance to think. In a positive example, we may see someone we love and we smile and are filled with loving feelings before we have a chance to think about it. However, we can also have negative emotional reflexes, commonly called triggers, in which someone or something causes a person to feel angry or upset before they have a chance to think about it. In order to free ourselves from negative emotional patterns, we must reprogram our "emotional reflexes" so our mind does not continue to *automatically* experience unwanted emotions. This is important when working through your Symptom Emotion or NPP, because if you are automatically experiencing these emotions before you have a chance to think, then you will never succeed at making the genuine and *lasting* change that is needed to heal yourself. And as much as we may want to, we typically cannot simply force ourselves to change.

To illustrate this, we can continue to build on this example of the ball being thrown at you. Let's say you make the conscious decision to try not to move and instead let it hit you in the face without any reaction. Could you do it? Likely, doing so would feel impossible. Why? Because it would not feel *safe*, and you are programmed to react. The same is true with your emotional reactions; you have programmed reactions. And if you want to respond differently you must reprogram your subconscious mind to do so.

THE 4 CATEGORIES OF MIND-BODY-SOUL-SPIRIT NEEDS

During my research, once I found evidence that we needed certain emotions for optimal health, I continued to search for any other emotions that we physically needed. My criteria were simple. I looked for emotions that most or all human beings would *innately* strive for, even without conscious thought. I also looked for emotions that would trigger irrational behavior and/or make people immediately reactive. For example, feeling "unsafe" may trigger a reaction, whereas feeling "unsure" typically does not. Although the distinction may seem insignificant, consider the contrast: imagine if you feel very unsure of what you are doing this weekend. Then, imagine if you feel very unsafe about this weekend. The latter could trigger a stress response due to our inherent need for safety.

I also found it helpful to study the automatic behaviors of children in order to gain clarity as to what was truly innate. Doing so began to reveal another need. It's well-known that if children don't get positive acknowledgment/attention, they might automatically engage in a negative behavior such as acting out, getting in trouble, or wanting sympathy.[10] The fact that children would rather gain negative attention/acknowledgment over being ignored indicates the level of importance that our subconscious mind places on these feelings as well as our innate drive for them.

Similarly, there are also well-documented attention-seeking behaviors in adults. These can include both positive and negative behaviors. On the positive side, individuals may seek achievement, rewards, or recognition for their good deeds. On the negative side, they may seek sympathy, superiority, or dramatic situations. This Need can be as simple as desiring acknowledgment for our efforts in daily activities, such as cooking dinner, or for ongoing efforts such as striving to excel in our professional endeavors. From this, we can see that human beings possess an innate need for acknowledgment and can unconsciously fill this need in positive or negative ways. Similar to safety and love, research has also documented that there can be a biochemical release in connection to attention, recognition, and reward.[11]

After extensive research, I found one additional emotion that we need. It is a bit different than the rest, however, it met my criteria of occurring without conscious thought. This one had to do with the feelings of *deserving*. I began to notice a pattern: that we only allow ourselves to have, feel, or experience what we subconsciously feel we deserve. Thus, if we don't feel deserving of something, we are likely to automatically and without conscious thought either not allow ourselves to fully enjoy it or sabotage our efforts to get it.

In many cases, people may not even realize they are sabotaging themselves. Such was the case for Sofia, whose painful ankle injury derailed her endeavors because she felt she did not deserve the success.

From this research, I developed the four categories of Mind-Body-Soul-Spirit Needs. They are:

- Safety and security
- Love and bonding
- Attention, acknowledgment, and reward
- Deserving, or being allowed

I named these needs the Mind-Body-Soul-Spirit Emotional Energy Needs because as I began to understand these Needs from a holistic and spiritual perspective, I noticed something fascinating. The four categories of emotions seemed to directly correspond to the four main aspects of humans: mind, body, soul, and spirit. It was as if each of these parts of us had a corresponding emotion that it needed. For example:

- **The Mind Need** (attention, acknowledgment, reward). When thinking of the most basic need of the mind, we can think of reward and ego. This can include anything that *feels* rewarding, including any benefit, attention, acknowledgment, or recognition.
- **The Body Need** (safety and security). If we did not have an innate and automatic drive toward circumstances that make us feel safe (such as not falling off a cliff), it would be hard to stay alive in our physical bodies. So it makes sense that we have an automatic drive toward that which makes us feel safe.

- **The Soul Need** (love and bonding). Our soul has a need for love, belonging, and bonding; these emotions are "food for the soul" and can trigger the release of positive hormones and chemicals that fuel our happiness and health.
- **The Spirit Need** (deserving or being allowed). This represents the connection between our physical body and life-force energy (Nature, God, Universe, Divine, etc.). In order to inhabit this body, we must, on some level, feel deserving of life and/or feel that we are allowed to receive from life. This fundamental need serves as a gateway to what we permit ourselves to receive or what we deny ourselves.

MIND-BODY-SOUL-SPIRIT
EMOTIONAL-ENERGY NEEDS™

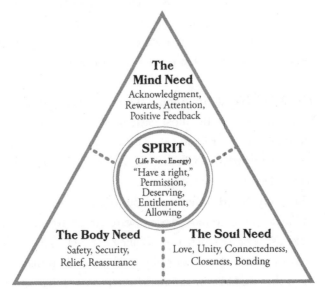

Exercise: Bring Subconscious Miswired Links into Your Conscious Awareness

Now that you have a basic overview of how these MBSS Needs work, it will be important for you to identify how these may be affecting your NPP, Symptom Emotion, or health. In the coming pages, we'll take a deeper look at each of the four MBSS Needs. As we do, I will prompt you with questions to help you identify information that may be unconsciously affecting your health. As we go through this process, you will begin to see just how counterintuitive and miswired our mind programming can be because we do not consciously create it. For that reason, I will share with you some examples, and then provide you with a series of questions you can ask yourself.

My goal in sharing these examples will be to "jog your mind." Even if you don't directly relate to the given example, reading it can assist your mind in bringing subconscious connections to the forefront of your awareness so you can free yourself from them.

Before we begin, there are a few things you will want to keep in mind:

- **Take your time to read through each of the four categories of MBSS Needs.** As we go through each example, notice if any of these types of thoughts or subtle emotions come up that are connected to your Symptom Emotion, NPP, or another negative emotion that you are working to free yourself from. As you'll recall, emotions that are illogical and subtle still matter. This typically means they are buried in your subconscious mind.

- **Vanishing Consciousness.** When you bring these subconscious links into your mind, you may quickly forget them if you don't write them down. This may sound odd, but they can be fleeting—here one minute and gone the next. This is what I refer to as "vanishing consciousness"— becoming aware of subconscious information which then vanishes. You may have experienced this in other areas of life if you have ever woken up from a vivid dream and you felt like you *absolutely* would remember it, but later you couldn't recall it no matter how hard you tried.

  It is extremely likely that you will experience vanishing consciousness at some point during this process of healing yourself and working with your subconscious mind. For this reason, it is vital to take notes of any valuable insights that come to mind for you. Otherwise, there is a chance that you'll forget them. At the end of the chapter, you will use your notes to begin the process of freeing yourself and then transforming these negative links in your mind.

- **Utilize the Freedom Techniques.** As always, and throughout this entire process, your goal is to stay in the positive as much as possible. This holds true as you go through this chapter. If any of your insights make you feel stressed, be sure to pause and implement the Freedom Techniques. Then, resume the process once you feel ready.

THE NEED FOR SAFETY AND SECURITY: THE BODY NEED

In many ways, the need for safety is the easiest MBSS Need to understand and see around us; however, the challenge is that in many cases we've learned to invalidate our fears instead of reprogramming them. As you'll recall, I made that mistake. Since I did not feel that my fears were valid, I ignored them. To avoid making that mistake, I'd encourage you to approach this exercise with an open mind.

Diego's example below may not directly apply to you, but it can help you to understand miswired MBSS Needs and get you thinking about your own MBSS Needs.

After reading the example, you'll begin the self-inquiry process. You'll want to keep it simple and focused, making sure not to dig up every negative emotion you've ever had. Instead, notice if your subconscious mind feels that your Symptom Emotion or NPP is keeping you safe.

An Example of Self-Criticism Being Linked to Safety: Diego

Diego had suffered from recurring headaches for more than ten years. Each time he got a headache, it would last for days. Following the steps of the GIFT Method, he worked to identify his Symptom Emotion, which turned out to be self-criticism. This was a pattern he'd been aware of and had been attempting to rid himself of for many years, but to no avail. However, as he used the Freedom Techniques outlined in Chapter 12 to begin shifting his feelings of self-criticism, he was able to release the pain from his headache. To his amazement, he even stopped getting daily headaches.

Diego was so ecstatic about his results that he stopped following through with the rest of the GIFT Techniques. After all, his pain was gone, and he didn't consider himself to be an emotional person, so he didn't see the need. At that time, Diego didn't realize how important it was for him to fully release the negative emotional pattern. Unfortunately, his old emotions of self-criticism soon returned, and so did his headaches. He restarted the GIFT Method, but this time he followed through with this step. This enabled him to see the reason that the pattern and pain came back: they were linked to his MBSS Needs. In short, Diego began to see that his subconscious mind was programmed to feel that self-criticism was keeping him safe. This is because he had grown up feeling constantly criticized by his father and, unbeknownst to him, his subconscious mind erroneously linked up that if he criticized himself first, it would keep him safe and stop others from criticizing him.

To break free from the pattern of self-criticism that Diego had for so many years, instead of struggling against his own mind, he needed to reprogram his subconscious mind that self-criticism was not actually keeping him safe. As Diego analyzed his Safety Need, he gained a clearer understanding of how his subconscious mind had linked self-criticism (his Symptom Emotion) to keeping him safe. Here is a list of illogical emotions that Diego found linked up in his subconscious mind:

- Diego's mind linked up that criticizing himself would keep him safe by protecting him from being criticized or yelled at by others. This pattern repeated in his life.
- Once Diego's mind linked up that self-criticism was keeping him safe, it became his "emotional reflex." Then, anytime he did something wrong or felt that someone was upset with him, he would automatically criticize himself. This was how his mind was programmed to keep him safe and avoid fear and danger.
- It felt unsafe for Diego to *not* criticize himself.

From this, we can clearly see the reason why Diego struggled to break free from this pattern: it was connected to his MBSS Needs in several ways. In this part of the process, you'll want to notice if you have similar subconscious programming linked up to your Symptom Emotion or NPP.

Common words/emotions that are used to describe this Body/Safety Need are:

- Safety (physical or emotional)
- Security
- Relief
- Avoiding fear (real or imagined)

Questions to consider about your Body/Safety Need:

- On a scale from 0 to 10, how safe/unsafe do you feel in life?
- On a scale from 0 to 10, what level of safety/fear do you feel toward your future?
- Do you subconsciously feel that your Symptom Emotion, NPP, or other negative emotion is keeping you safe?
- Do you feel that you will be unsafe if you let go of your Symptom Emotion, NPP, or other negative emotion you are working on?
- If you identified any miswired programming, jot it down so you can transform it in the coming steps. If analyzing these questions brought up negative emotions for you, be sure to shift them before proceeding. To do so, you could utilize: the Freedom Techniques to release negativity, the Step G Techniques to lift your emotions, and Power Writing to create a list of reasons that make you feel safe, so you can then amplify those feelings.

THE NEED FOR LOVE AND BELONGING: THE SOUL NEED

When it comes to the emotions that fuel the energy of the soul, this category can include feelings of connectedness, such as love, bonding, nurture, affection, and feeling included. However, like the other MBSS Needs, the need for love can get erroneously linked up to unhealthy emotions, in which case we can block ourselves from receiving it. For example, a person can feel that it is not safe to love, and therefore avoid love.

Other ways this MBSS Need can negatively affect our health is if we erroneously get love linked up to our Symptom Emotion, or NPP. The problem is that these miswired links can be completely counterintuitive.

An Example of Depression Being Linked to MBSS Needs: Alicia

Alicia, a devoted wife and mother of three young children, had been struggling with depression. Despite her belief that she shouldn't feel this way, she was plagued by a persistent heaviness.

Alicia began to explore her MBSS Needs to understand why her mind was holding on to these negative emotions. She paid attention to her subtle emotions and realized that if she were happy, she'd feel selfish. As a mother, she felt that the right thing to do was to put herself last. Therefore feeling happy also triggered feelings of guilt. While these emotions had always been there, Alicia hadn't realized it. Consciously, she did not want to feel this way. However, she could see these emotions were connected to her MBSS Needs in several ways:

- Alicia knew her husband loved her, but she was surprised to find that a part of her feared losing intimacy with him if she were happy. After all, he had always been the most nurturing on her darkest days.

- She felt that if she were happy, she would not fit in or be able to connect with her friends.
- Because Alicia's friends and family were going through difficult times, part of her felt that they would judge her if she appeared to be too happy. She also feared losing their love and support.

Alicia knew these feelings were illogical, and because they were subtle thoughts, she previously would have ignored them. However, as she began to understand her MBSS Needs, she realized these thoughts were indications of the deeper programming that was in her subconscious mind. Unconsciously, her mind was prioritizing meeting her emotional needs of safety and love. However, due to miswiring, her mind was programmed to believe that being happy would result in losing safety and love. This kept her stuck in a state of depression.

You'll want to notice if you have any miswired mind programming that is linked up to your Symptom Emotion or NPP.

Common words/emotions that are used to describe the Soul/Love Need are:

- Love
- Unity
- Bonding
- Relating to others
- Feeling included
- Intimacy
- Nurture

Questions to consider about your Soul Need:

- On a scale from 0 to 10, how loved do you feel in life? How unloved do you feel?
- On a scale from 0 to 10, how much do you feel that it's not safe to love others or to be loved?
- Do you feel that your Symptom Emotion or NPP is subconsciously programmed to help you gain love or keep you from losing love?
- If you found miswired programming, you'll want to write it down. If analyzing these questions brings up negative emotions for you, be sure to shift them before proceeding. To do so, you could utilize the Freedom Techniques, Step G Techniques, and Power Writing to begin lifting your emotions and amplifying positive feelings of love.

THE NEED FOR ATTENTION, RECOGNITION, ACKNOWLEDGMENT, AND REWARD: THE MIND NEED

We all have a need for acknowledgment, attention, and rewards. This can be met in simple ways such as: a compliment from your spouse, acknowledgment for a thoughtful act, a child wanting you to watch them ride their bike, or even receiving an award at work. These emotions drive us at a subconscious level and are vital for our happiness and well-being. As we discussed previously, these emotions can even trigger the release of positive biochemicals in our bodies.

At first glance, some people may feel an aversion toward this particular need, perceiving it as ego-driven. However, it is important to remember that we can fulfill this need in humble and loving ways. When this need is met in positive ways, it can fuel our happiness and health.

Many people have a combination of both positive and negative subconscious patterns connected to this need. The problem is that most are unaware of these patterns. Instead, the pattern may appear as an unfortunate life circumstance. For instance, imagine a person who has a negative experience and receives attention for it (in the form of sympathy) or feels like a "good person" in a victim scenario. Although they may not consciously want to feel this way, their brain can link these positive feelings of attention or love to the negative experiences. This programs their mind that negative events can fulfill their positive needs. For this reason, even when a person wants to release the negative pattern, they can't fully let it go because part of their mind feels like it meets their needs. Furthermore, if we consider repetition compulsion, we can see how this painful pattern can repeat and continue to resurface in a variety of different ways that may appear unrelated.

An Example of Miswired Mind Need: Nisha

Imagine the case of a little girl, Nisha, who experiences rejection from a group of girls her age. She is then told by a loving adult, "Don't worry. They're just jealous. You're better than they are."

While this is meant to be a thoughtful gesture, it's important to remember how the mind works. It is likely that due to this comment, Nisha will experience feelings of attention, superiority, or righteousness and inadvertently link those feelings up to the initial painful feeling of rejection (not because it's logical, but because the two events occurred at the same time).

She may unwittingly continue to attract repeated circumstances where she feels rejected, along with feeling righteous or superior. (Refer to the Emotion-Perception Cycle on p97.) Likely, she will start to see herself as being superior and develop a pattern of fault-finding in others to show her mind that these people who are rejecting her are inferior. This can cause her to be condescending or exude an attitude of superiority over others without consciously realizing it, which will likely result in more rejection and perpetuate this pattern.

This painful Rejection/Superiority Pattern might continue throughout Nisha's life in a range of different ways:

- She might grow up, have an argument with her family, and experience feelings of rejection. As a result of her pattern, she will likely tell herself that she is superior and that her family is just not as smart, good, spiritual, or evolved as her.
- She might experience ongoing feelings of rejection from an event. For example, she may feel upset that her ex-boyfriend cheated on her, yet she may hold on to those feelings and feel superior over him because she was good enough to forgive him.
- She might feel an ongoing sense of rejection from men because she is single, or she may feel that her husband doesn't pay her enough attention. Due to this subconscious pattern, she may mistakenly feel it's because the people in her life are inferior, not mature enough, or have another fault. This will again repeat the pattern of feeling both rejection and superiority.

As you can see, this can be a very painful cycle, and it's very common. The Rejection/Superiority Pattern often starts with a miswired Mind Need but can ultimately get erroneously linked up to several needs.

Common words/emotions that are used to describe the Mind/Acknowledgment Need are:

- Attention
- Acknowledgment
- Accolade/Reward (verbal or material)
- Pride/Good
- Special
- Unique
- Recognition
- Emotions commonly connected to the ego

Questions to consider about your MBSS Mind Need:

- On a scale from 0 to 10, how much do you feel that you receive positive attention?
- On a scale from 0 to 10, do you feel it is safe and good to get positive attention?
- Do you feel that your Symptom Emotion, NPP, or negative emotions are gaining you attention (even if you don't consciously want the attention)?
- If you found miswired programming, you'll want to write it down so you can change it in the upcoming exercises. Then make sure to return to your positive programming to reinforce positive feelings that it is safe and good to get positive attention. You could use Power Writing to list positive ways that you currently fulfill this MBSS Need or have met this need in the past. Then make a point to *feel* positive attention and acknowledgment.

THE SPIRIT NEED FOR
FEELING DESERVING

The best way to think of the Spirit Need is to look at what you specifically feel that you are allowed, permitted, or entitled to have or experience in life, and what you feel you need to do in order to deserve this.

When many people first hear the word "deserving," they might immediately and mistakenly think that it has to do with feeling unworthy or not good enough. But that is not the case. Since this mistake is extremely common, let's hone in on the difference. The subconscious rules for deserving can be the *opposite* from feeling not good enough or unworthy. For example, one person may feel they are not good enough and subsequently feel as though they *don't deserve* to receive from others. Yet another person may have the opposite belief and *feel* that because they are not good enough, it means they are incapable of doing things for themselves. As a result, they feel they *deserve* to be taken care of by others.

While it is common for people to confuse "deserving" and "worthy," they are distinctly different emotions that work in a very different way. For example:

- I have worked with people who grew up with several siblings and an overwhelmed single parent. This resulted in developing feelings of scarcity toward love; they felt there was not enough love and attention for everyone. In these situations, a person may believe that the sick child deserves love and attention, feeling it would be selfish to receive it themselves. This example illustrates how a person can feel worthy of something yet not feel that they deserve it. Moreover, they may feel worthy but guilty for receiving it. When it comes to healing, the distinction is both simple and profound.

- This MBSS Need can also control your Symptom Emotion, NPP, or any other negative emotion. For example, if you feel that you *deserve* to be angry, it can feel impossible to fully release feelings of anger until you change this programming.

- This is also true for feelings of self-punishment, as was the case for Diego. Since he grew up with criticism from his father, at a young age he developed a belief that if he made a mistake, he deserved to be criticized. To successfully change this pattern, he had to program into his mind that humans can make mistakes, but he did not deserve to be berated for his mistake. Instead, he deserved an opportunity to try again. This was very different programming for Diego, which helped him to finally free himself from his Symptom Emotion that had plagued him for so long.

Common words/emotions that can be used to describe this Spirit/Deserving Need are:

- Allowed to receive
- Entitlement
- Having a "right to"
- Having permission

Questions to consider about the Spirit/Deserving Need:

- On a scale from 0 to 10, how much do you feel you deserve to have a happy, healthy, and enjoyable life?

- On a scale from 0 to 10, how much do you feel you deserve to get attention and love?
- Do you feel that you deserve your NPP (e.g., deserve punishment or deserve to punish or take from others)?
- Do you feel that you "have a right to" feel your Symptom Emotion (e.g., a right to be angry, upset, or hurt)?
- On a scale from 0 to 10, how much do you feel you deserve to be punished for your past actions?
- If you found miswired programming, you'll want to write it down so you can change it in the coming exercises. You'll also want to make a point to reinforce your feelings of deserving by implementing the Give Yourself Permission exercise (p172). As you do the exercise, you can use the word "permission" as we originally discussed, or you can use the word "deserving" if you'd prefer. Use whichever wording feels best to you, or both. As you do, really feel into it so that you have strong feelings that you deserve a happy, healthy, and wonderful life.

An Example of Physical Illness Being Linked to MBSS Needs: Johnny

In some cases, a person's mind can become miswired leading to a subconscious belief that illness is necessary for safety or to fulfill another one of the MBSS Needs. For example, I worked with a boy named Johnny who was being picked on by two boys at school. He became so nervous and fearful about going to school that he began suffering from stomachaches daily. Since he was sick, he had to stay home where he felt safe and protected. Because there were strong emotions connected to this experience, Johnny's subconscious mind unintentionally linked up that he needed to be sick, as it was the only way for him to stay home where he was safe.

It may sound odd that the mind could make this connection. However, as discussed earlier with the example of self-harm, in certain situations, the mind can be wired to attack or harm the body if it perceives safety or benefit in doing so. The subconscious mind, as you know, is not rational. It doesn't analyze stored information but associates things that occurred simultaneously.

Johnny was stuck vomiting on and off for about eight months and seemed to have one random health issue after another. During that time, he was placed on several different types of antibiotics which didn't resolve the issue. No one could figure out what was wrong with him, especially considering that his symptoms continued to change.

Every time Johnny went to school, he experienced extreme feelings of fear and would vomit. He would then be sent home where he would experience feelings of safety and love, which, after happening several times, created a link in Johnny's mind, unbeknownst to him, that he needed illness to keep him safe and loved. Johnny's mom helped him overcome his fear. She showed him online that even his favorite superhero movie had negative reviews, which surprised him. She used this to reassure him that he didn't need to be hurt by others' words but instead to have compassion for them, as they were stuck in a critical mindset. She also told him that if he didn't let their words bother him, they would stop. Naturally, she kept a close eye on him and asked his teacher to do the same. It was a remarkable success; Johnny experienced feelings of security and confidence that had an immediate impact. His health issues vanished, and he returned to school. The boys who used to tease him stopped. In fact, he became friends with one, and the other got transferred to a different class.

I share this example of Johnny because it's easier to understand how this information can get unknowingly linked in a child's mind. And like any other pattern, it can also repeat itself. This means that if you have had recurrent illness in your life, there is a chance that your subconscious mind has associated it with safety or fulfilling one of your other MBSS Needs, even if you don't consciously believe it's true.

In fact, when Diego went through my course to work on healing himself from his headaches, he was initially surprised to find that his mind had linked up self-criticism to safety. And then he was further surprised when he found that his mind had also linked that his headaches kept him safe and even got him love. As a child, when he was sick, this was the only time his dad was loving to him and wasn't hard on him. Obviously, he didn't want to feel this way consciously, or he would not have been taking my video course. However, as with the example of self-harm, our minds can become miswired more than we realize, but not because it is intentional.

Questions to consider:

- Do you feel unsafe to move forward in life for any reason, or do you feel like someone is beating you up, including yourself? If so, this can create a "Johnny" situation of fear.
- Do you feel that any of your MBSS Needs have been subconsciously linked to illness?
- Do you feel that people who are sick seem to receive more of the MBSS Needs?

If you have answered "yes" to any of these, you will want to write them down. In the next chapter, we'll focus on transforming any miswired or unhealthy MBSS Needs you identified so you can reprogram your mind to help you step into the happy and healthy life you deserve. It's crucial that your subconscious mind can meet its needs in positive, healthy ways, so let's work on that first.

Reinforce and Fulfill Your *Healthy* MBSS Needs

As you read through this chapter, if you've noticed that any of your MBSS Needs are not being met or are being met in unhealthy ways, then it will be important to ensure that you're fulfilling them in positive ways.

To do this, you'll want to:

- Review your notes from the self-inquiry process. If you notice that any of your MBSS Needs are not being met (e.g., you have been feeling unsafe or unloved), or they are not being fulfilled in healthy ways (e.g., your way of connecting with others is through illness or hardship), then write them down. You will want to prioritize fulfilling these needs in positive, healthy ways.
- Write down a few positive ways that you'd like to meet these needs. Use your favorite Step G Techniques to visualize and experience meeting these needs in healthy ways. Do this for any of the MBSS Needs you wrote down in the last step.
- Once you get clear on how you want to feel, as always, you'll want to use the Step G Techniques to access and amplify your emotions.

Now that you know the importance of these MBSS Needs, you'll want to reinforce your positive MBSS Needs toward being both happy and healthy.

- Use Power Writing (p173) and jot down all the reasons why healing will increase safety, acknowledgment, and love. Also, list the reasons you truly deserve to be happy and healthy. Even though your conscious mind may know all of these things, the more you energize these positive emotions in your subconscious mind, the more it can help you speed up your results. Your Power Writing list could include some of the following:
  - o Being healthy and happy will enable me to feel more loved in life
  - o Being healthy and happy will enable my partner/spouse and me to have a lot more fun together
  - o I deserve to have a healthy and happy life – we all do
  - o Being healthy and happy will attract more love, as people are naturally drawn to those who radiate positivity and overall well-being.

Note: Even though this may seem simple, it will be important to program this into your subconscious mind. If you've been injured for a long period of time, you may have found yourself feeling jealous or envious of those who are happy and loved, which can inadvertently link up these negative emotions to being healthy and happy, albeit subconsciously. Or you may have told your mind that you don't even want to think about the fun things you could do if you were healthy. While this can be understandable, this way of thinking can keep you stuck. However, the more you can energize your mind and emotions about how wonderful it is to be healthy, the more it can help you to speed up your results.

- Now that you know your mind will automatically fulfill these MBSS Needs, even in unhealthy ways, practice implementing positive changes into your daily actions, even in little ways. Make a point to connect with people in positive ways and abstain from meeting your MBSS Needs in negative ways, such as such as engaging in self-criticism, etc.

By now you know the importance of these MBSS Needs, so before moving on to the next chapter, make sure that you have thought of several healthy ways in which to meet your needs. Keep following through to program this information into your mind so you feel these emotions intensely! In Step T, we will begin the transformation and release process.

Summary of the Key Exercises in This Chapter

- Set aside your notes from the self-inquiry process; we will use them in the next chapter. Remember to prioritize programming your positive MBSS Needs first.
- Implement the "Reinforce and Fulfill" Process to fulfill any unmet MBSS Needs and to help accelerate healing. Follow through for at least 30 days or until they become your new norm, whichever is longer.
- Continue using the Step G Techniques daily and utilize the Freedom Techniques as needed to reduce and release negative emotions.

STEP T OF THE GIFT METHOD: TRANSFORM

In this step we will focus on:

- Applying the step-by-step release process
- Transforming yourself for a healthy and happy self-image to promote self-love and self-healing
- Releasing, reprogramming, and transforming any negative patterns you have identified
- Factor 5 of the 5 Factors for GIFT Mind-Body Healing

This step includes:

Chapter 14
Transform, Reprogram, and
Release Unhealthy Emotional Energy

Chapter 15
Transform Your Health and Uplift Your Life
Through Positive Embodiment

STEP T

14

TRANSFORM, REPROGRAM, AND RELEASE UNHEALTHY EMOTIONAL ENERGY

We are what we repeatedly do. Excellence, then, is not an act, but a habit.

—Will Durant[1]

Welcome to the Transformation Step! Here you'll find a detailed process to help you create a radical shift for each of the 5 Factors that you've identified, including your Symptom Emotion, NPP, and any miswired MBSS Needs you have uncovered. As you reprogram and release old, unhealthy mind programming and embrace the transformation, you can align your body with its natural state for self-healing.

Take your time! You won't want to rush to complete this step because it would be too much to reprogram everything at one time. If you're feeling rushed, then logically the feeling that will get programmed into your mind is the feeling of "rushing" because that's how you *authentically* feel. It's that simple.

With that in mind, it will be best to take your time and keep your focus on authentically feeling differently, and follow through all the way so that you *fully* shift your emotions and your perspective. This is key for radical healing to occur.

A FEW IMPORTANT NOTES

Before diving in, you'll want to do a self-check to ensure that 1) you are still following through with your Step G Techniques every day, and 2) you have begun to master your ability to lift your emotions.

It is common for people in our culture to hold a strong belief that as soon as we release negativity, we will be filled with happiness. But that's not how our minds actually work. That would be akin to thinking that if you suddenly stop speaking English, you'll know how to speak French. Logically, you will not know how to speak French unless you learn it, program it into your mind, and practice it. The same is true with new emotions.

If you have not yet become proficient at programming in your new Positive Emotional Patterns from Step G, then you'll want to get in more practice before proceeding with the transformation and release process. If you have already become skilled at programming in positive emotions and you are ready to proceed, fantastic! Here are a few things to keep in mind:

- Each and every time after you work with your negative emotions, you'll want to end the process by using the Step G Techniques to ensure you keep your emotions lifted.
- Notice the emotions you're experiencing. You can't trick your mind and nervous system. How you genuinely feel matters. As you make your way through the upcoming process, you must do so in a way that feels uplifting, fun, and expansive. If you feel as though you're going down memory lane or wading through painful memories, then you'll want to stop and focus on the positive before proceeding.
- If at any point you start feeling unpleasant, overwhelmed, or have an increase in negative emotions, then it's a sign that you most likely have unresolved NPP. If this happens, you'll want to revisit the list of NPP on p164 to ensure that you're not trying to justify any actions or intentions that are not in complete spiritual integrity.
- Remember to never "hang out" in your negative emotions. If you find yourself doing exactly that or berating yourself for them, then it would be best to take a break from the book—to give yourself space from working on yourself—and resume only when you're willing to be kind to yourself and move forward in a *positive* way.

Before we dive in, I want to share a quick example of the release and transformation process so that you have an idea of what to expect.

An Example of the Release and Transformation Process in Action: Andre

When Andre came into my class, it wasn't hard to tell that he was feeling depressed. It turned out that he used to pride himself on being a happy, healthy, and positive man, but that had changed eight years earlier when his wife died. After she passed, he fell into a deep depression. Over the next few years he began struggling with one health issue after another. One week his back would hurt, the next his legs, then his feet, knees, shoulders, and so on. As Andre put it, he felt as though he was falling apart.

Once Andre began exploring his MBSS Needs, he was able to see that his wife's death had dramatically changed the way he operated in life and how he was meeting his MBSS Needs. He was surprised to discover that deep down he felt that if he were happy, people (including his grown children) would judge him and think that he didn't love his wife or that he was glad she was gone. Further, he felt that if he remained upset and in mourning, then people would think he was a good man. This was exactly opposite of the way that he wanted to feel consciously.

As he analyzed these thoughts, he could see that throughout the years, several people had even complimented his mourning, saying or implying that it signified an obvious devotion to his wife.

Probing his MBSS Needs even deeper, he began to see that he also felt guilty for the idea of having a good time without his late wife, as well as guilty for the fact that she was the one who had died rather than him. After all, she had always been more health conscious than he was; therefore it didn't seem fair.

Now that you are familiar with MBSS Needs and also NPP, you might be able to see the problem: even though Andre consciously *wanted* to be happy, based on his miswired subconscious mind programming, happiness didn't meet any of his MBSS Needs.

Below are examples of how Andre's mind was miswired regarding his MBSS Needs towards both happiness and mourning.

Happiness:

- Happiness evoked guilt. (NPP and Spirit/Deserving Need)
- He didn't feel that he deserved to be happy. (Spirit/Deserving Need)
- If he were happy, he felt that he could be judged. This did not feel safe. He felt as though he could lose love. (Body/Safety and Soul/Love Needs)

Mourning/Depression:

- If he were mourning, he felt proud that he was a good husband who had loved and cared for his wife. (Mind/Acknowledgment Need)
- He felt that while being in mourning, he received an outpouring of compassion and love from friends and family. (Soul/Love Need)
- He felt that if he were no longer mourning, people would go on about their lives, leaving him lonely and forgotten. This did not feel safe. (Body/Safety Need)
- Deep down he felt that the right thing to do was to keep mourning. (Spirit/Deserving Need)

As you can see, your mind does everything for one reason: it is programmed to do so. Based on Andre's miswired mind programming, happiness did not feel like it met his MBSS Needs, so his mind *automatically* wanted him to stay away from happiness. Mourning and depression were meeting his MBSS Needs, so his mind automatically wanted to hold on to these emotions.

This was the opposite of what Andre consciously wanted. As he became aware of his miswired MBSS Needs, he could see the reason that it had felt so hard for him to be happy and the reason that everything he'd tried to do hadn't worked. With that, Andre began reinforcing his positive MBSS Needs (Chapter 13) and began to genuinely feel that being happy did meet his MBSS Needs.

Then, using the steps in this chapter, he began working to reprogram his mind, starting with his NPP (guilt). As he worked to release the feelings of guilt and undeserving from his subconscious mind, he immediately felt lighter and life moved with greater ease. After he felt the authentic shift occur, he gave himself a few days to practice and experience these new feelings. Then, once he was able to genuinely feel the shift, he moved on to reprogram both his future expectations and then his past trauma.

I will share additional insights from Andre's transformation in the coming process; however, there are a few points to keep in mind:

- Make sure that you have already reinforced your *positive* MBSS Needs (Chapter 13).
- If you have a pattern of guilt or any other NPP, you'll want to address that pattern first.
- The *order* of Reverse Emotional Processing is important (p94). Andre needed to reprogram his current mind programming first before addressing his future and past wounding.

As Andre followed through each day to reprogram his subconscious mind, his life continued to transform. He experienced deep feelings of happiness and laughter again, his aches and pains completely vanished, and he felt more alive and in love with life than he'd felt in years.

Now it's your turn.

Transform Miswired MBSS Needs

Release Technique 1

In this first exercise, it will be important to reprogram your MBSS Needs that are connected to any negative patterns you have identified throughout this process. As an example, if you have a miswired negative emotional pattern, such as self-criticism that is linked up to feelings of safety, then your goal in this exercise will be to reprogram that completely so you are able to shift your emotional patterns in the same way that Andre did.

You can use this process to reprogram any of your negative patterns, including your Symptom Emotion, or any other negative emotional pattern keeping you from achieving continuous Positive Expectation and Optimism. You can also use this process if you noticed that your MBSS Needs were directly linked to your illness.

As we begin, it's assumed that you were already able to discover at least one—and likely several—miswired MBSS Need(s) as you went through Chapter 13. However, if for any reason you were unable to, don't worry. Skip ahead in this chapter to p290 to the exercise called "Did You Overlook Anything?" Then, once you've identified an emotion, come back here to this exercise to begin reprogramming your mind.

- First, select a pattern to release (I suggest your NPP or Symptom Emotion). Apply all three release techniques in this chapter to that emotion. (After you complete the process, return here to work on your next pattern.)

- Identify any MBSS Needs that are connected to the emotion you chose. (Refer to your notes from Chapter 13 or Andre's example on p273.)

  Here are a few examples of miswired MBSS Needs that we've discussed:

  o Andre felt acknowledged for being a good husband for staying in mourning. He even received an outpouring of love and compassion from his grief even though he didn't consciously want it.

  o Diego felt that he deserved to be criticized and also that self-criticism kept him safe.

- Next, implement the Emotional Brushing Technique (p228) toward the negative emotional pattern, along with any miswired MBSS Need links connected to it. Using Diego as an example, he'd want to brush down toward, a) the feeling of criticizing himself, b) the feeling that self-criticism kept him safe, and c) the feeling that he deserved to be criticized.

- Next, you'll want to get clear on your New Positive Replacement which is the new programming for your mind. (Note: this step is similar to your 180° Shift. The 180° Shift represents the "big picture shift" you've used until now. However, now that you know your MBSS Needs, in this step you'll refine the details to include them so you can effectively reprogram your mind.) To do this, you could start by asking yourself two questions:

Question #1: *What do I want my mind to automatically do instead?* Write down your new replacement.

Example with Diego:

o Instead of being self-critical, I will treat myself with kindness, love, and support.

o If I make a mistake, I will lovingly support myself and correct the issue, if possible, and then learn from it and move on.

Question #2: *How does this new way of thinking, feeling, or acting meet my MBSS Needs even more than the old pattern?* List all the reasons you can think of. (This can help create new positive MBSS Needs.)

Example with Diego:

o By treating myself with kindness and support, I will feel more confidence and happiness, which is also much safer for my health.

o This is a much *safer* way to proceed. I will feel better about myself, which will also feel safer and promote more love in my life.

o In proceeding this way, others will *respect* me even more, which will result in more *loving* connections.

o The more I treat myself with kindness and loving support, the more I will be able to experience more *love* for myself and for others.

o The more I am kind and supportive to myself, the more it will help me flourish and live the loving, *rewarding* life that I *deserve*, as we all do.

o I deserve to treat myself with support and kindness. We are human, and we all make mistakes. I deserve to kindly support myself so I can flourish in life and in love.

Notice in Diego's list, he includes the very things he wants in life and also covers all four categories of MBSS Needs. You'll want to do the same.

- Next, it's important to reinforce your New Positive Replacement along with your new MBSS Needs, to get them fully programmed into your subconscious mind. To do this, you can use your favorite Step G Techniques.

  Using Diego's example, he could get a Power Vision of himself experiencing the new feelings from his list. He could step into his vision using Visual Reality and use the NT Music Technique to help him repeatedly access and reinforce these new feelings of safety. For an example, as an NT Music Technique song, he could use the song, "I'm Good" by the Mowgli's to take in the feeling that he is good, then read his list of new MBSS Needs and really *feel* it!

- Next, you'll want to get your mind to deprogram the negative pattern. To do so, you can implement Constructive Negative Mind Programming. As the name suggests, this means we will incorporate a touch of negative mindset programming. This may sound contradictory, considering that we have thoroughly discussed the impact of negative emotions and the importance of eliminating them. However, let me provide you with a quick example to illustrate the reason this exercise is crucially important.

Imagine a two-year-old in the kitchen near a hot oven. The toddler's loving mother points to the oven door and calmly repeats, "No. Hot. Ouch. Don't touch. Ouch." From this, the toddler gets it linked up in their mind that it's not safe to touch the oven. The toddler may repeat, "Owie. Hot." This is an example of constructive negative programming and training your mind what *not* to do.

However, there is a very important detail to notice in this example: The mother does *not* take her child's hand and put it on the oven door and burn her child or yell at them in order to teach them. Doing so could be traumatic and harmful for the child's health and happiness. Regardless of age, you don't need to be yelled at or be hard on yourself in order to learn, but you will need to get new programming into your mind—both positive and negative.

Many of us learned all sorts of things in a similar way from our parents when we were growing up. We all learned that it would be painful to get hit by a car or fall off a cliff, and yet we didn't need to personally experience these things to get this programmed into our minds. Instead, our parents said, "Watch out! A car is coming!" or "Get down from there! You're going to fall and hurt yourself." As a result, this information became programmed into our subconscious minds. To this day, if a car is driving toward us, we have a *reflex* reaction to automatically pay attention and quickly move if needed.

This type of constructive negative programming is important in mind programming because your mind must have clear direction about what you do and don't want it to do. After all, you would not want to hike up a mountain and have your nervous system be flippant about falling off the mountain. That would be bad programming! Moreover, you definitely would not want your mind to think that in order to stay safe, it would be good to fall off the cliff! Obviously, that's not safe. While this scenario may seem ridiculous to imagine, I use it to emphasize the point that our emotions can be extremely illogical.

After all, Diego's mind had been programmed that self-criticism was keeping him safe. If this programming remained in his subconscious mind, it would have been nearly impossible for him to stop criticizing himself. Therefore, he would not have been able to heal himself. For this reason, it was imperative for Diego to reprogram his mind and understand that continuing to criticize himself was unsafe.

To implement Constructive Negative Mind Programming, Diego made a list of reasons it was unsafe to continue criticizing himself. With consistent follow-through, his subconscious programming changed. As a result, his mind stopped automatically attacking (criticizing) himself.

This is the importance of Constructive Negative Mind Programming—to get your mind to deprogram old patterns. Without deprogramming, it can feel hard or impossible to change. In fact, if you have listened to my podcast, you may have heard me nudging people a bit to change for this very reason: Your mind must stop taking its old path.

You will need to get it programmed into your mind that the old way *does not* meet your MBSS Needs. Since your mind has been following the old path for so long, if you do not clearly program into your mind that the old path is unsafe, it will likely continue to take the same route. In this case, you may not achieve tangible results.

To implement this, you'll want to make a point to specifically *invalidate* any of your old miswired links to your MBSS Needs.

Constructive Negative Mind Programming
Example: Diego

- I now see that criticizing myself is not safe. It has caused me physical pain. It attracts more criticism into my life and is a horrible pattern to be stuck in. If I keep criticizing myself,

I will not be able to feel truly confident and good about myself, which will mean less love and acknowledgment, and a loss of safety.

- I used to think I deserved to be criticized if I made a mistake, but I now realize everyone makes mistakes; we are human. I don't deserve to be criticized, and it is not safe to think in this way. Instead, I *deserve* a chance to learn from my mistakes and grow from them, just like everyone else.

As you can see from these examples, Diego wrote down all the reasons why his negative pattern would ultimately hinder his ability to meet his MBSS Needs.

You'll want to do the same so that you can begin deprogramming your miswired MBSS Needs. Make sure your list is convincing and motivates you to want to change. When you read this list each day, keep in mind that unlike other exercises, you will *not* be focusing on bringing in as much emotional intensity as possible. Instead, referring back to the example of the toddler with the oven, you'll want to make it clear to your mind that the old path is "ouch" (unsafe), but you don't need to "burn yourself." Your goal is to reprogram your mind instead of being mean to yourself or feeling horrible.

With that in mind, you'll want to write these statements in a way that feels *constructive*. If you have a strong personality, you can write things to push yourself a bit to change, as long as they *feel* inspiring and motivating, not painful. If you have been feeling sensitive, you may not want to push much at all. Use your intuition to gauge how far to push yourself and do whatever makes you *feel motivated and inspired* to change.

So far, in summary, you will have:

- Identified the miswired MBSS Needs that are linked to the negative pattern
- Implemented the Emotional Brushing Technique toward the miswired programming
- Decided on a "New Positive Replacement" and how it will meet your MBSS Needs
- Used the Step G Techniques to begin programming this into your mind
- Implemented the Constructive Negative Mind Programming Technique to program into your mind that your negative pattern is not meeting your MBSS Needs, and that the pattern is painful so that your mind will fully release it
- Remembered to end on a positive note by returning to your Step G Techniques, including your Power Vision(s) and any 180° Shift to keep your mind focused on the positive.

Now that you have gained clarity of the process and the specific changes you want to program into your mind, you will want to make sure to reinforce this new mind programming at least three times a day for 30 days, or until it becomes your new automatic way of thinking and feeling. To do so, you'll want to read through these exercises with a focused intention and desire to embrace this new way of thinking and feeling. The more you can continue to *decrease* and *release* the old emotions connected to your miswired MBSS Needs and get yourself amped up to use the new positive mind programming, the easier and faster it will be to shift into your new positive mindset.

Note: Before moving on to the next exercise, it would be wise to take a few days or more to embrace and embody this shift as much as you can. In the next exercise, we will continue working with the same pattern but in a different way.

Transform Your Life and Future

Release Technique 2

As you may have experienced, if you're getting rid of an old household item, it can be difficult to throw it away if you think you might need it again. Similarly, I have found the same to be true with our emotional patterns. If any part of our mind expects that we will need the pattern in the future, it will not want to let it go. Furthermore, this expectation can become programmed into our mind without us ever realizing it. This is because our mind can automatically assume that if a problem occurred in the past, it is likely to recur. Then, despite our best attempts to clear negative patterns, our mind may still hold on to the negative emotion because it expects to need it. The purpose of this exercise is to address and release those hidden negative expectations.

To do so:

- On a scale of 0 to 10, ask yourself how much you expect a negative situation to occur that might require your old pattern. If your answer is a definitive 0, then great! You can simply skip the rest of this exercise and move on to the next. But if you notice that even a small part of you expects it to happen again, then you'll want to continue.

- Next, knowing that strong emotions can shift your perception, utilize Power Writing to create a radical shift. List the reasons you are confident the problem won't recur. Embrace positive expectations and feel it!

- Use the Freedom Techniques toward your negative expectations so you can start eliminating them. While implementing this exercise, if a specific negative situation comes to mind that you expect to recur, then you'll want to shift it. To do so, write down the reasons you could expect a more positive situation or outcome in the future. With follow-through, this can help shift your expectations.

Note: In the next exercise, we will continue working with the same pattern but in a different way. However, before doing so, it would be wise to take a few days or more to embrace this shift as much as you can. Taking this approach can make the next steps even more effective and help set you up for success.

Transform the PEST: Clear Past Programming

Release Technique 3

In Aimee's situation, you'll recall that her pattern of feeling unloved began in her childhood with her father. Then it continued into her relationships and marriage. As you know by now, our patterns can continue to repeat. For this reason, it will be helpful to identify when your pattern became stuck in your mind, so you can release it completely.

As we work through this process, there are some key details that you'll want to implement that are different from the norm. You may have already worked on childhood trauma; however, in this case, instead of looking for a pattern in general, it would be advantageous if you can be more specific and look for the first time this issue was linked to your MBSS Needs.

This is what I refer to as the Past Emotional Seed or Trauma (PEST)™. I define it as the first time this emotional pattern was "seeded" into your mind along with any MBSS Needs. This will be important because the patterns that end up repeating themselves are almost always the ones that are in one way or another connected to your MBSS Needs. To begin releasing this PEST, you'll want to:

- Think back to the very first time you remember experiencing the negative emotional pattern that you're working to clear. If you can't remember the exact time, don't worry. You can simply try to recall the *feeling itself* from the earliest time that you can remember and work with that.
- As you think of the first memory, notice if any of your MBSS Needs are being met in that situation. For example:
  o In Aimee's case, when her father ignored her, her mother kindly made a point to give her extra love. While this was a very nice gesture, this linked love to the pattern of feeling unloved. I understand this may sound counterintuitive to many people. But remember the subconscious mind does not analyze information. That's not its job. The subconscious mind stores information much like the hard drive on your computer. And when two things occur at the same time, they can get linked up, regardless of whether we want them to or not.
  o In Nisha's case, you'll recall she was left out, and the consoling adult at that time helped her to feel special and superior. This linked up rejection to feeling superior.
  o In Andre's case, shortly after his wife's passing, he'd had a moment of feeling happy, immediately followed by guilt

and concern of what others would think. He also had
the pattern that it was good for him to feel guilty, which
began in childhood.

o   In Diego's case, when he was a child and his father was
criticizing him, he found that his dad would stop if he
criticized himself. This made him feel as though self-
criticism kept him safe.

• Next, implement the Emotional Brushing Technique toward
the pattern as well as any and all MBSS Needs you identified
in that memory.

Note that the negative pattern can get linked up to different
MBSS Needs at different times. For example, safety may get
linked up to the pattern at age four while love may get linked up
at age seven. Be patient with yourself and work on one thing at
a time so you feel empowered instead of overwhelmed.

• Next, invalidate the miswired MBSS Needs that are linked
to the PEST. To do this, use the Emotional Brushing
Technique and simultaneously remind your mind that
the pattern is not meeting any of your Needs. (Similar to
Constructive Negative Mind Programming, p280, you'll
want to be willing to shift your perspective.) As you follow
through, you may notice that the memory fades away.

In my own life, no matter how hard I try, I cannot find my old
negative patterns from my injury. They feel similar to having
had a belief in Santa Claus as a young child. Sure, I know that
I used to believe in Santa Claus, but I no longer relate to those
feelings, and they do not feel true to me. I have a completely
new perspective. Much like there is no part of me that is going
to get sucked back into that old perspective of believing there is

a grown man who can fit down a tiny chimney, my old patterns no longer make logical sense to me, and I no longer feel they are true. I now see that I was simply caught in a pattern. Your goal will be to feel the same way about your negative patterns.

- As you work to bring in the new perspective and use the Emotional Brushing Technique to let go of the negative emotions, your memory of the PEST can start to dissolve and/or change for the positive, automatically. Using the same example as before, Nisha might start to see herself as a young girl playing harmoniously with other children, or the old memory may disappear completely. Optimally, you want the memory to change on its own or disappear entirely so that none of the old emotions remain. However, if the PEST memory does not automatically dissolve or change in a positive way for you, then no worries; you'll want to transform it for yourself as you work through the rest of this process.
- Using the same example as before, Nisha can envision her younger self feeling completely secure and at ease around other children. In her vision, she could feel a sense of love and joy when playing with them, feeling included and valued as an equal. It's important to include all four categories of the MBSS Needs in your vision. Make a conscious effort to repeatedly reinforce this programming, allowing yourself to embrace a new way of feeling genuinely.
- Be sure to notice the absence of the old negative emotions. For instance, there are no feelings of rejection or superiority in the transformed memory. Be willing to embrace the transformation.

- It's best to do this exercise daily for at least thirty days, or until you have genuinely cleared and transformed the PEST from the past, and your new, positive way of being feels completely natural and automatic.

Optional Additional Step: When we discussed Emotion-Controlled Perception in Chapter 7, I mentioned that people will often work with their younger self from a wounded state of mind. If you have previously done that, then it is possible you may have accidentally and unknowingly *reinforced* negative patterns instead of *released* them. Don't worry. This is quite common and can be correctly reprogrammed using the steps on p290. While there are several reasons this can happen, I want to warn you of two of the most common mistakes that I've seen.

First, as people work with their childhood wounding, they may feel sorry for their younger self. While this may be understandable, this can further ingrain unhealthy emotions like self-sympathy. This emotion can be linked to health conditions and since emotional patterns tend to repeat themselves, can also get stored in the subconscious mind and repeatedly manifest unwanted circumstances (situations that make you feel sorry for yourself). If you have done this, I would recommend using Release Technique 3 (p284) to release and transform these feelings. Then make a point to feel impressed with yourself.

Second, the other most common mistake I have witnessed throughout the years is that a person may recall a time they felt wounded, hurt, or lonely as a child and then, in an effort to heal the problem, they may give their childhood self a hug or extra love in that moment. However, now that you understand your MBSS Needs, you may be able to see the problem with this. It links up the problem emotion with even more love, which can inadvertently fuel the pattern to continue showing up in your life in a variety of different ways. Therefore, as you work with your childhood self in this step, you'll want to be careful not to do this. If you have done this in the past, don't worry. You can simply use the Emotional Brushing Technique toward those negative emotions as well.

If you want to instill additional feelings of love into your younger self, try this exercise. Recall a time when your younger self acted positively—kind, loving, good, smart, or fun. Make a point to love and acknowledge your younger self for this. If you can't remember a specific memory, simply envision your younger self exhibiting the positive qualities that you would like to reinforce in your current life. To do so, you can simply use visions that include feelings of being loved, safe, deserving, or included, etc. Then amplify these feelings to the best of your ability. If you have experienced a challenging childhood, consider incorporating this exercise into your daily routine to further amplify these emotions.

If you realize that you have inadvertently reinforced a negative emotion in the past, or if you grew up feeling like you were severely lacking any of your MBSS Needs, then I would highly recommend following through with this extra exercise for the next thirty days.

I mentioned previously that we would be processing our emotions in a different way and in a different order (Reverse Emotional Processing, p94). For that reason, I understand this release process may seem like a lot to learn. However, once you get the hang of it, it can become faster and easier to implement. At this point, take a moment to reflect on your changes.

Then, when you feel ready, if you have additional patterns that you want to release, you will want to go through the same process to address those as well, starting with the "Transform Miswired MBSS Needs: Release Technique 1" exercise on p275.

Did You Overlook Anything?

Questions to Help You Bring Hidden Subconscious Links to the Surface

As you know by now, there can be multiple layers of emotions that are connected to a negative pattern and/or illness. For that reason, it would be good to double-check that you didn't overlook any hidden links that may keep you stuck.

I've created a list of questions to help bring your awareness to any additional links that could potentially be affecting your 5 Factors for GIFT Mind-Body Healing. You'll want to uncover all the links you can in order to *fully* activate your body's natural self-healing mechanism.

As you read through the questions, notice what comes up for you. If at any time you are able to gain clarity on a pattern needing transforming, it's best to stop reading the list at that point and then work to transform the issue before proceeding. This is to ensure you are processing one thing at a time without overwhelming yourself. In this case, you would simply want to write down your new insight so you don't forget it and then refer to Release Technique 1 on p275.

You can also use the Emotion Contrast Technique (p166) to gain clarity of any remaining feelings that may be buried in your subconscious mind.

- Even if I know I don't consciously want _____ [insert Symptom Emotion/NPP, negative emotional pattern or health issue], does it make me feel safe, loved, special, unique, good, and/or deserving in any way?
- If I did not have this _____ [insert Symptom Emotion/ NPP, negative emotional pattern, or health issue], would

I feel *less* safe, loved, acknowledged, special, or deserving in life?

- Have I been holding on to any feelings of self-punishment?
- Do I find myself justifying my actions?
- Do I frequently feel alone or lonely? Do I avoid people?
- Do I feel loved, nurtured, special, or cared for having _____ [insert Symptom Emotion/NPP, negative emotional pattern, or health issue]? (Even if you don't want it, is the feeling there?)
- Do I find myself frequently talking to others about my illness or connecting with others who are either sick or have similar negative emotional patterns?
- Do I find myself using _____ [insert Symptom Emotion/NPP, negative emotional pattern, or health issue] as an excuse to either get out of obligations, or as a "hall pass" so I can do something I want instead?
- Do I feel like I take breaks or do nice things for myself only when I am sick?
- Have I found myself feeling jealous of others for getting attention from their illness? Did I get it linked up as a kid that people who are sick deserve more attention?
- Do I feel afraid, fearful, or worried about my life in the future?
- Do I have an intention to take from others or do I want to get revenge on someone who hurt me?
- Do I feel like it's 100 percent safe to be healthy today, right now? (As odd as it may sound, many people futurize the possibility of getting better, saying things like, "I'll get better in a month," or "I'll get better after I do such and such." *Now* feels too soon. If you notice this, you will want to change it so that your answer is, "Yes! I feel ready *right now!*")

- Do I feel that sickness is keeping me from addressing something I'm afraid of? For example, on numerous occasions, I have worked with people who wanted to get better and have told themselves, "As soon as I get better, I will start dating, or [go do such and such]." Yet deep inside, they actually have a fear of the future activity. Subconsciously, their bodies do not feel it is safe to heal, prioritizing their short-term *emotional* well-being over their long-term *physical* well-being.
- Do I have a behavior that blocks me from connecting with others, such as being angry, abrasive, passive-aggressive, fault-finding in others, jealous, or having social anxiety?

As you read through this list of questions, if you noticed that you still have additional patterns to work on or multiple patterns, make sure not to overwhelm yourself. Instead, simply focus on the pattern that you intuitively feel pulled toward or the one that impacts you the most since it would likely have the biggest benefit.

Also, remember to be kind and loving to yourself. This can help you more easily embrace these changes in your mind programming. Then, you'll also want to embody these changes into your daily actions to complete the transformation, which is what we will be working on in the next step.

Summary of the Key Exercises in This Chapter

- Take your time going through each part of the process. Be sure to follow through with each step completely and immerse yourself in the positive changes until you develop a new automatic way of thinking and feeling.
- To the best of your ability, strive to maintain a state of Positive Expectation and Optimism each day until it becomes your new normal.
- Continue using the Freedom Techniques daily, as needed. Also, do your best to refrain from engaging in negative emotions and situations until you have fully healed yourself.
- Be sure to follow through with your new mind programming for *at least* thirty days after you have healed yourself. In short, go *beyond* the goal!

15

TRANSFORM YOUR HEALTH AND UPLIFT YOUR LIFE THROUGH POSITIVE EMBODIMENT

Every action of our lives touches on some chord that will vibrate in eternity.

—E.H. Chapin[1]

It's common in our culture for people to fall short of making lasting changes in their lives because they never change their subconscious mind programming. This can be most easily observed when people set New Year's resolutions for changes they want to make. Unfortunately, most never realize that in order to create lasting change, they need to change their mindset to establish new ways of thinking and feeling as well as new physical habits. For these reasons, many people may fall short of making the changes they desire.

Conversely, the opposite can occur: You can work to reprogram your subconscious mind, but if you never allow yourself to fully integrate the changes into your actions and behavior, these changes may never become part of who you are. That is the importance of this chapter: to learn how to embody the changes into your daily actions so you can make a genuine transformation. After doing so, you'll need to update your self-image so that you see yourself as being happy and healthy, feeling genuinely good about yourself and loving who you are! That will complete Factor 5 of the 5 Factors for GIFT Mind-Body Healing.

THE FOUR Cs FOR CHANGE

To make it easy to incorporate the changes, I've created the Four Cs for Change, which are four key points that will be important for setting yourself up for successfully transforming your habits, actions, and your daily life. They are:

1. **Clarity**. Gain clarity about how your negative patterns may have influenced your unconscious actions and identify what you are going to do differently.
2. **Commitment**. Follow through consistently until you establish new habits.
3. **Courage/Confidence**. Take real action.
4. **Celebration**. Acknowledge your successes along the way, whether big or small, to reinforce long-term changes.

As you read through each of the Four Cs, I encourage you to have a quiet place to think and write. As you contemplate each one, you'll want to write down a few ways you can apply the information in your life so you can work through the process as we go.

If at any point you are unsure of what to do, the best way to figure it out would be to imagine someone else in your shoes. Give them your best advice to set them up for success. Then take it for yourself.

1. Clarity

In this first C, your goal will be to get clear on how your *actions* may be unconsciously fueling the negative pattern. When we discussed the Emotion-Perception Cycle on p97, I mentioned that in many cases when you have a negative emotional pattern, your actions may be unconsciously fueling the problem.

For example, in Diego's life, after he began reprogramming his patterns of self-criticism, he began to see with more clarity where these patterns had shown up in life.

He recognized that he frequently felt criticized by his boss. While he'd always been successful at work, he observed with a newly opened mind that he was often late and frequently missed deadlines. Previously, anytime his boss mentioned the issue, Diego had always defended his actions or had an excuse for them. However, once Diego began clearing his patterns, he realized this was a major source of the criticism in his life. He was grateful for the clarity because he could finally see that this was not who he wanted to be in life and he was not fully in integrity.

To apply this in your own life, you can simply think about each pattern that you are getting rid of and ask yourself where it shows up in your life. This can help you gain clarity about any problematic behavior or actions that may be fueling the negative pattern. This may pertain to an NPP, Symptom Emotion, or any unhealthy MBSS Need linkage.

Now that you have clarity on a problematic action or behavior that you want to change, it will be important for you to get clear on what you want to do differently and then commit to that change.

2. Commitment

Commonly, when people decide to discontinue a certain behavior, they may simply tell themself to *"just stop doing it."* However, this does not typically work. Instead, you'll want to commit to a new way of being that you can turn into a new habit.

Referring back to Diego's situation, he decided to do two specific things differently:

- To ensure he arrived on time, he committed to leaving ten minutes earlier for work each day.
- When it came to project deadlines, he made a point to get better at managing his time.

To create lasting change, it is crucial for you to make a dedicated commitment to consistently follow through. By doing so, you can establish new habits that will positively impact your life. For example, Diego decided that he needed sixty days to truly establish his new habits. During that time, he made a commitment to both of these actions: arriving on time for work every day and meeting all of his deadlines.

You'll want to do the same in your life. To implement this:

- First, consider your old behavior and then decide what new action you are willing to commit to so that you can begin to embody the changes.
- Second, decide what length of time you are going to commit to so you set yourself up for success in creating a new habit.

As Diego followed through and embraced change, he was able to completely free himself from his debilitating headaches and gained a new level of self-confidence. He then went on to create his next Power Vision, which included buying a house and getting married. He then began taking steps toward doing exactly that. To his delight and surprise, both came to fruition. Approximately two months after creating this vision, he met a woman. The following year they got married and bought a house together. These were things that he had dreamed of doing for many years. However, once he was willing to change his mindset and his actions, they became his reality.

From this we can see that when you follow through—even with seemingly small, new daily actions that are in alignment with your new positive mind programming—it can have an enormously positive impact on your life. To make a plan, ask yourself, *For how long am I going to follow through with my change? How frequently?* You can also include any additional details, such as the time of day, etc. Do whatever it takes to set yourself up for success.

I would recommend initially setting a commitment time of between thirty and sixty days, with the goal of following through every day so that it becomes automatic, like brushing your teeth.

When you get to the end of your goal date, check in with yourself. If your desired new positive actions have become automatic daily habits, great. If it does not quite feel automatic yet, it would be best to add another thirty days.

3. Courage and/or Confidence

As you put your desired changes into action, you may realize that even small changes can require courage. This can be particularly true if you've been injured for a long period of time.

To help you build courage, create a list of reasons why you know you can achieve what you are wanting, and the reasons you want it today. Ensure these reasons are strong, and read them daily. This can help build your confidence and motivate you to step out of your comfort zone to make it happen. For example:

- *If others can do it, I know I can too.*
- *I don't want to wait another ten years. I am ready to do this today.*
- *If I follow through, I know I can do anything.*
- *I have succeeded at other things in life, so I know I can do this.*
- *I can see that I am changing, and I expect life to get better and better.*

You can use these ideas to get started, and of course, feel free to list as many more reasons as you can. The more, the better. As you read them each day with emotional intensity, you will notice your feelings of confidence and courage increasing, which can be transformative.

You could also write down examples of past successes in your life to remind yourself of how amazing you are, which will continue to build the confidence and conviction that you are the one who holds the power to transform your life for the better—but it's up to you to use this power!

4. Celebration

As you know by now, your subconscious mind loves benefits, rewards, and acknowledgment. So as you follow through with taking new positive actions in your life, you'll want to reward yourself in healthy, positive ways. Maybe you could treat yourself to a massage or simply take a moment to authentically acknowledge yourself and really feel it.

It would be best to choose a variety of rewards—ideally both small, daily rewards for "little wins," and bigger, long-term rewards. For example, one man in my program set up a celebration dinner with friends and family when his doctors told him that all of his tests came back clear. Continuing to follow through, he set up another celebration dinner when he reached one hundred days of being healthy and going for walks outside each morning—something he could not have done previously. One thing I love about his story is that he engaged his family in his celebration. He began having regular family dinners, making a point to celebrate his children's and wife's successes too! This was a beautiful uplift for his health and his entire life.

I've seen people set up all kinds of celebrations, from trips to fun destinations to parties with friends and family. Please celebrate in whatever way feels good for you, as recognizing your successes can help lead you to even more success.

Align Your Actions with Your Mindset Using the Four Cs

It's now time to review what you have written for the Four Cs for Change and to make sure that you have set yourself up with a successful plan.

First, carefully read through the information you wrote down for each of the Four Cs, then write down anything you feel may be missing from this plan or any changes you feel need to be made.

Next, on the same page, write down all the benefits to making these changes. Be sure to include anything positive and exciting and, of course, any way that it will help you meet any of your underlying MBSS Needs.

Place this written list next to your bedside so that every morning when you first wake up, you can take just a minute or two and read it to help you immediately get your mind on track to embody the changes.

As you follow through to make these changes in your actions and behavior, you'll also want to continue with your internal mind programming from the previous chapters. As you embrace these changes, you'll be creating the new healthier, happier, version of yourself. Then it will be important to ensure that your mind has a view of you that is in line with this newly transformed you.

THE IMPORTANCE OF UPGRADING YOUR SENSE OF SELF-IDENTITY AND SELF-IMAGE

Your sense of self-identity and self-image is your mind's blueprint of you; it's the way you see and feel about yourself and what you are capable of. As you step into the new happier, and healthier you that you've been working to create throughout the GIFT Method, it will be crucial to update your self-image to include your new positive patterns. This will help you to solidify the positive changes you have been starting to make and to embody your overall positive transformation. If you don't do this, you may well find yourself inadvertently starting to slip back into your old, negative patterns and be unwittingly held back by your outdated perception of yourself.

For example, if your Symptom Emotion was a longstanding pattern of being self-critical, there's a chance that even if you've transformed the old, negative emotional patterns, you may still see yourself as being inferior or in some way "less than." It's important to update, or upgrade, your self-image to one that will allow you to continuously feel positive about yourself and experience genuine self-love.

It will also be of utmost importance to make sure that you picture your "new" self as someone who is 100 percent healthy. This is particularly important if you've been injured or sick for a long time, or if you've ever identified as being "just like" a friend or family member who is (or was) often ill, as your mind may still subconsciously see yourself as a "person who is sick," which could actually end up making your body subconsciously want to keep or recreate illness if you don't shift it.

In the exercise that follows, you'll learn how to up-level your self-image to feel all-round happier and healthier and genuinely love who you are. Doing so can help uplift many areas of your life simultaneously and bring about real, lasting healing.

Upgrade Your Self-Love and Self-Image: The Positive Self-Reflection Technique

Before we begin the steps of this exercise, there is an important distinction that I want to note. There is a difference between seeing yourself *acting* in a new way versus *seeing* yourself in a new way. To be successful with this exercise, you'll need to focus on the latter: seeing yourself in a new way.

Because so many people tend to get these confused, I want to carefully illustrate the difference using a simple analogy. Imagine for a moment that you are looking at a painting and you are fixated on everything that you don't like in the painting, but you are trying to force yourself to genuinely love it. How would that go? Likely you would not experience genuine feelings of love for this painting.

Now, continuing with this analogy, imagine that you start releasing your negative emotions toward the painting and make a conscious effort to notice the aspects you genuinely like about it. Every day, you focus on these positive elements, allowing yourself to truly love them and making a point to really feel it. As a result, you find yourself falling in love with this painting and seeing it in a new light.

In this exercise, you are the painting.

- Close your eyes and visualize yourself in an imaginary mirror. See yourself as being happy, with a big, beautiful smile on your face. You are glowing from within. Your shoulders are relaxed and back, and you are feeling healthy and happy.

    (You can also try this with a real mirror if you'd like. You may find that to be helpful or you may find yourself feeling the need to look perfect, which could be distracting. As always, do whichever feels best to you.)

- In your imaginary mirror, make a point to see yourself standing tall, feeling happy, confident, and smiling. Take a few moments to really absorb what it *feels* like to see yourself in this new way and to be this new you.

- Now shift your focus to purposely feel those exact same emotions within your own physical body. You might feel a big smile emerging on your face, as if your body is glowing and radiating with health and happiness from within. (Keep in mind Emotion-Controlled Perception; the more you can amplify these emotions, the better!)

- Now practice alternating between two exercises: First, observe your new, positive self in the mirror and note the emotions it evokes. Second, immerse yourself in these emotions, feeling them deeply. This practice can help you reprogram the way you see and feel about yourself!

- Build on this exercise by imagining or "pre-picturing" this new, positive version of yourself walking around in places that you frequent, such as your house. Then actually walk around your house in the same way, feeling like this new, healthy, happy version of yourself.

Another idea is to do this in a public place, like the grocery store. Before you go to the store, take a moment to pre-picture the new, healthy, happy version of yourself walking around inside, doing your shopping. Notice how you feel about this new version of yourself in your vision. Then, once you actually go into the store, notice what it feels like to walk around being this new version of you. Feel it.

- As you walk around, you'll want to feel like the new you, seeing yourself healthy and genuinely embodying your 180° Shift and the positive changes that you have been working on throughout this process. Thoroughly feel good about yourself and honestly love who you are.

- As with every other exercise in the GIFT Method, a combination of repetition and bringing in strong positive emotions are key. Be sure to do this exercise every day for at least thirty days until your new, positive sense of self-identity feels like your new norm. This is typically when I witness healing occur: when individuals address their MBSS Needs, NPP, and Symptom Emotion, while also maintaining a state of Positive Expectation and Optimism. Witnessing people heal themselves in this way has become a regular part of my life. That is my hope for you—that you embody real change and turn any illness around by tapping into the extraordinary innate power that we all have to heal ourselves.

Summary of the Key Exercises in This Chapter

- Continue to follow through with your daily GIFT mind-programming exercises to create a real transformation. Keep in mind that genuine change is key.
- Implement the Four Cs so that you can genuinely transform your life.
- Use the Positive Self-Reflection Technique to increase feelings of self-love and embrace the new, happier, and healthier you!

SO, WHAT NOW?

Congratulations! You've reached the end of the GIFT Method.

"What now?" you might ask. Well, it all depends on what you've found along the way and where you are with your daily work and your results so far. By this point, you may have already been able to release your pain or observed other noticeable changes in your health, and you've fully healed yourself. If so, fantastic! You'll want to remember to celebrate your successes.

If you're not there yet, that's okay too! You'll want to celebrate your success for making it here to the end of the process. Then make sure to keep yourself excited and motivated each day so that you can get yourself to fully follow through. One way to do that would be to listen to my podcast and enjoy the inspiration of witnessing others shifting their pain in real time. Since you now know the method, you'll understand why it works.

People often ask me how long it takes to activate the body's self-healing mechanism. There's no simple answer to this, as it takes different amounts of time for different people in different situations with different health issues and other individual factors.

In my experience, the biggest factor leading to success is one thing: embracing real change. Upon doing so, I've witnessed people heal themselves completely in very short periods of time.

An example you can hear on my podcast is an interview with a woman who'd had a tumor in her throat for several months.

She'd tried everything she could think of in an effort to get her body to heal naturally, but it was not working, so she was scheduled to have it removed via surgery. However, through an interesting turn of events, she and I connected the day before her surgery. In a last-ditch effort to heal herself, we had a session where I coached her through the steps of the GIFT Method.

When she woke up the next morning, she could no longer feel the tumor. She assumed it must have moved. However, when she went into the hospital for her scheduled surgery, her doctors were perplexed. They had just taken the latest MRI of the tumor a few days prior, yet now they couldn't find the tumor. It was gone! Her surgeon said he had never seen anything like it in his thirty years of practice.

In order to heal herself, she had to let go of some old hurt that had been weighing her down. As she did, it was life-changing! She felt liberated and empowered to do the things she'd been wanting to do, including opening a new tea company, which she proceeded to do. She now has a tea company that ships organic tea around the world!

While I have worked with a few others to achieve similar results, her speed of healing was obviously much faster than you would typically expect for more serious issues such as tumors. Most people simply aren't able to embrace change quite as rapidly. However, this particular client had been extremely determined to transform her mindset, emotions, and actions and began doing so within minutes of understanding the changes that she needed to make to heal herself.

I completely understand that for many people her story may sound impossible. So if you'd like to hear more and watch a short video after she left the hospital, you can find this information and an interview with her on the website for this book. You'll also want to note that even though she took charge of her own healing, she did not avoid her doctors. You'll want to be sure to do the same and continue to work with your doctors.

Others who have gone through my courses have been able to use their minds to do incredible things, like go from being bedridden to moving, walking, and even running! Of course, in these situations their successes took longer than one day. It's not a race; you will want to go at the speed that feels best to you. That was the case for another woman who went through my program. She had been diagnosed with an extreme case of POTS (postural orthostatic tachycardia syndrome), Mast Cell Activation Syndrome, as well as a variety of other health issues, including chronic pain and extreme food allergies. Due to her health challenges, she was not able to eat easily and therefore had to start the healing method very slowly, so her transformation to health was not overnight. She was able to reduce her pain within the first month and gradually began to add foods into her diet. However, it took about nine months for her to heal herself in full—after which, all her medical tests, including her EKG, came back normal for the first time in thirteen years. Less than three months later, she walked her first 5K, renewed her driver's license, and began to travel around the world. You can learn more about her story on the website for this book, too. My point in sharing this is to emphasize that you'll want to go at your own pace. More importantly, as you do, make sure to embrace real change.

I'm very thankful to say that on a daily basis, I see people manifest healing results that most others would consider miracles. As I am writing this, I just received an email from a woman who joined my program to heal herself from rheumatoid arthritis. In her message she expressed awe that the pain in her hands was completely gone after only a couple of weeks since starting the program. It had been five months of being pain-free and she couldn't believe it. She is elated to be returning to her job in technology after having been unable to work for three years.

From the range of examples given here, I hope you can see that the time it takes for each person to activate their body's self-healing mechanism varies greatly, depending on how fast they are able to embrace and implement real change in relation to each of the 5 Factors for GIFT Mind-Body Healing.

So where are you on your path to healing, and what should you do now?

- If you have healed yourself already—great! I would recommend that you keep following through for at least an additional month to make sure your new, positive mind programming feels like your new norm and that you have completely released your unhealthy mind programming.
- If you've identified and worked to lessen your NPP, Symptom Emotion, unhealthy MBSS Need link, or any other negative emotion, and you're starting to notice positive changes and/or you feel better (whether a little or a lot), then excellent! Keep going! And keep in mind that to achieve real, tangible results, you must make a real, radical shift in your emotions so that you are genuinely feeling elated each day. If you hear your mind saying, *I will be happier after I heal*, you'll want to remember that is backward thinking.
- After I healed myself, many people initially thought I was so happy *because* I had healed. However, it was the other way around. I lifted my emotions so much and released any negativity, and as a result, my body healed. Every

day I feel deeply grateful that I took the time to do so. That said, if you are not yet genuinely feeling like you are glowing and in love with life, you'll want to make sure to embrace real change.

• If for any reason you've only read the book and have not put any of the techniques into practice yet, or you have not fully followed through to see improvement, then you'll want to go back and work to implement each step to its fullest so that you can begin to connect with your innate abilities to heal yourself and uplift your life.

In summary, when it comes to the amount of time it will take to heal, the more you're willing to embrace real change, the sooner you can tap into your body's fullest potential to heal itself. That's when the magic happens. But remember, going faster doesn't always help to achieve faster results; real change does. You must genuinely think and feel differently and see life in a new, more positive way. So go at your own pace; your goal is to embrace genuine change in order to make this life-changing!

A FINAL NOTE

You can probably tell by reading the stories in this book that I love people. I love working with people and teaching them to use their minds to connect with the spiritual essence of life that resides within us all. Maybe one day I will have the honor of meeting you in person, or connecting with you in an online workshop, and hearing your success story too.

I often get asked, "How is it possible that you're always so happy?" The answer is because I *programmed* myself to feel this way and embodied the change.

My sincerest hope is that you do the same—that you take from these pages what makes sense to you and what applies to you, then fully and consistently implement it in your life. Anyone can reprogram their subconscious mind, but it does require an honest effort and follow-through. Be willing to change, but also to be willing to fill yourself up and embrace each of your MBSS Needs so that you genuinely feel excited and optimistic about your life, as well as safe, loved, acknowledged, and important—because you are!

I also hope you know that you deserve to have a wonderful, happy, healthy, and loving life, because we all do!

If you feel the need for additional support, my hope is that you will reach out for it. At the time of writing this, I offer ongoing group support as well as online video courses that can further support you in your self-healing, as well as services in other areas of life that can be a source of stress, such as relationships and financial matters. Even simply listening to my podcast can help support you, as it can add new perspectives, depth, and breadth to what you already have learned. Whatever your needs may be, I want to be sure that you feel supported to achieve the results that you are intending.

Please remember that healing yourself isn't in any way about avoiding your doctor or other medical professionals. Make sure that your doctors know you're working with your mind, and have them continue to oversee your health and medications.

As you know by now, the power of healing with the mind and emotions has been written about throughout history. My hope is that this generation will bring this approach to healing more out into the open. And the best way to do that is to get real results! Each of us must truly learn to master our own minds and succeed at healing ourselves—making it the new normal way of living for the betterment of all and for future generations.

Research has shown that it takes approximately 20–25 percent of a population to reach a tipping point for large-scale change in terms of a transition in collective dynamics.[1] My hope is that you become part of that 25 percent. This means that the more you can follow through to get lasting results in your own life, the more it can help others for generations to come.

On that note, if you benefit from this book, I'd sincerely appreciate it if you'd recommend it to others who are still suffering: leave a review, show it to your loved ones, and tell others about it—even if you're not quite friends with them (yet!). Let's not leave anyone behind. Every person matters.

There's currently a shortage of physicians in many countries, and projections estimate that shortages will continue to worsen. For example, in the US alone, the Association for American

Medical Colleges (AAMC) reports that physician shortages could reach over 100,000 during the next twelve years.[2] In the UK, it's estimated that there will be a shortage of almost 10,000 medical professionals in the next ten years.[3] We cannot continue to let illness rise at the exponential rate it has been increasing in recent years. It's vital now more than ever to embrace the innate healing power that lives within us all. Let's be honest: Even if there *were* more than enough medical providers, who wants to spend their life sick and in pain? We *all* deserve a better life than that. And we all deserve to be and feel empowered in our own lives.

Imagine if every person in the world felt empowered and was able to embrace their happiest, healthiest, and best self.

This is my new Power Vision for our world.

This would transform the health and happiness of our world, as change really does begin inside each one of us.

As each person becomes empowered and learns to master their own mind, this contributes to a change in our world around us, allowing us to see new possibilities. Together, we can create a better world for us all.

THE GIFT METHOD: GLOSSARY OF TERMS

All marks are protected by trademark and copyright.

5 Factors for GIFT Mind-Body Healing. The five emotional-energy components that can contribute to illness in the body or block your body from healing itself. It is when you address each of these five factors that you can activate your body's natural healing mechanism. p71

Emotion Contrast Technique. A simple technique to help you become more aware of your subconscious emotions and distinguish between them by introducing something entirely new to contrast against them. p166

Emotion-Controlled Perception. The awareness that subconscious emotions can shape the way we see and experience life. p95

Emotion-Perception Cycle. The awareness that if we have an intense emotional pattern, our own thoughts, emotions, perception, actions, and beliefs can further increase the pattern ultimately keeping us in a cycle. p97

Emotional Brushing Technique. Freedom Technique 2. An exercise designed to help you reduce or release the negative emotions in both your mind and nervous system. p228

Freedom Techniques. Techniques you can use to help free yourself from unwanted emotions. p228

Mind-Body-Soul-Spirit (MBSS) Emotional-Energy Needs. Specific emotions and energy that we as human beings all need for optimal heath and healing. They are Factor 4 of the 5 Factors for GIFT Mind-Body Healing. p243

Negative Punishment Programming (NPP). Factor 2. Having patterns of actions or emotions that make us feel that, for one reason or another, we deserve punishment. p158

Neuro-Transformational Music Technique. You use music to repeatedly access and create the specific emotions that you want to program into your mind. p144

Past Emotional Seed or Trauma (PEST). This represents the first time a negative emotion was seeded into your mind, or became a trauma in your mind, along with any MBSS Needs that were seeded with it at that time. p284

Positive Expectation and Optimism. Factor 1. Getting strong feelings of optimism and positive expectation programmed into your subconscious mind. p89

Positive Emotional Patterning. Establishing new positive ways of thinking and feeling that become programmed "paths" (or patterns) in your mind. p119

Power Vision. A vision for your life that is short, succinct, and to the point. A key distinction of a Power Vision is that the emphasis will not be on the vision itself but on amplifying your positive emotions. p118

Power Writing. A writing technique to further amplify your positive emotions and get them programmed into your subconscious mind. p173

Reverse Emotional Processing. Processing your emotions in reverse order from the standard way by engaging only with positive emotions *first* before addressing negative emotions. p94

See Mind Technique. A shifting technique that can help begin to shift your mind away from that which you no longer want and gently guide it toward that which you do want in life. p232

Stress Interrupt and Freedom Technique (SIFT). Freedom Technique 1. An exercise designed to help you reduce or release the negative emotions by getting "distance" from the problem to increase mental clarity. p175

Symptom Emotion. Factor 3 of the 5 Factors for GIFT Mind-Body Healing. The specific emotion that is associated with each symptom or ailment. p183

Vanishing Consciousness. When you are becoming aware of subconscious information and then it suddenly vanishes. p248

Visual Reality Technique. To the best of your ability, making your body position and movements correspond with the positive emotions related to your Power Vision. p136

SOURCES AND CITATIONS

CHAPTER 1

1 Epigraph: The Best Liberal Quotes Ever: Why the Left is Right (2004) by William P. Martin, p. 173.

2 Stanford Medicine, "Complex Regional Pain Syndrome (CRPS)," Stanford Medicine website. Available at: https://med.stanford.edu/pain/about/chronic-pain/crps.html (Accessed: 21 Jan. 2023.)

3 Jeong S., An J. and Cho S. (2021). "Role of affective instability on suicidal risk in complex regional pain syndrome: a diary approach" (preliminary report), *Korean J Pain*, 1, 34(1), pp.94–105. Available at: doi: 10.3344/kjp.2021.34.1.94. PMID: 33380572; PMCID: PMC7783859.

4 Ibid.

5 Mayo News Releases (2013). "Nearly 7 in 10 Americans Take Prescription Drugs," Mayo Clinic, Olmsted Medical Center Find," Mayo Clinic website. 19 June. Available at: https://newsnetwork.mayoclinic.org/discussion/nearly-7-in-10-americans-take-prescription-drugs-mayo-clinic-olmsted-medical-center-find/ (Accessed: 21 Jan. 2023.)

6 Australian Bureau of Statistics. (2017–18). *Chronic conditions*. ABS. https://www.abs.gov.au/statistics/health/health-conditions-and-risks/chronic-conditions/latest-release.

7 Steffler, M., Li,, Y., Weir, S., Shaikh, S., Murtada, F., Wright J.G., and Kantarevic, J., *CMAJ* February 22, 2021 193 (8) E270-E277; DOI: https://doi.org/10.1503/cmaj.201473.

8 Health Promotion Board. Chronic Diseases-A Growing Problem in the Workplace. Last Updated: 06 Oct 2022. https://www.hpb.gov.sg/article/tips-to-prevent-and-manage-chronic-diseases-in-the-workplace#:~:text=Singapore's%20ageing%20population%20and%20adoption,high%20blood%20cholesterol%20%26%20stroke).(Accessed: 21 Jan. 2023.)

9 Hvidberg, M.F., Johnsen, S.P., Davidsen, M. *et al.* A Nationwide Study of Prevalence Rates and Characteristics of 199 Chronic Conditions in Denmark. *PharmacoEconomics Open* 4, 361–380 (2020). https://doi.org/10.1007/s41669-019-0167-7.

10 UK. Fit for Work? Half UK workforce could face chronic illness by 2030 https://www.ihc.co.uk/fit-for-work-half-uk-workforce-could-face-chronic-illness-by-2030/#:~:text=Fit%20for%20Work%3F-,Half%20UK%20workforce%20could%20face%20chronic%20illness%20by%202030,policy%20makers%2C%20employers%20and%20patients (Accessed: 21 Jan. 2023.)

CHAPTER 2

1 Epigraph: Marie Curie, Scientist & Nobel Prize Winner. Our Precarious Habitat (1973) by Melvin A. Benarde, p. v

2 Wilhelm, M., Winkler, A., Rief, W., Doering, B.K., Effect of placebo groups on blood pressure in hypertension: a meta-analysis of beta-blocker trials, Journal of the American Society of Hypertension, Volume 10, Issue 12, 2016, Pages 917–929, ISSN 1933–1711, https://doi.org/10.1016/j.jash.2016.10.009.

3 Freeman, E. W. *et al.* (2015). "Placebo improvement in pharmacologic treatment of menopausal hot flashes: time course, duration, and predictors," *Psychosom Med*, Feb–Mar; 77(2), pp.167–75. Available at: doi: 10.1097/PSY.0000000000000143. PMID: 25647753; PMCID: PMC4333078.

4 Lu, C. L. and Chang, F. Y. (2011). "Placebo effect in patients with irritable bowel syndrome," *J Gastroenterol Hepatol*, 26 April, Suppl 3, pp. 116–18. Available at: doi: 10.1111/j.1440-1746.2011.06651.x. PMID: 21751434.

5 Lidstone, S. C. (2014). "Great expectations: the placebo effect in Parkinson's disease," *Handb Exp Pharmacol.*, 225, pp.139–47. Available at: doi: 10.1007/978-3-662-44519-8_8. PMID: 25304530 https://pubmed.ncbi.nlm.nih.gov/25304530/.

6 Benedetti, F., Carlino, E. & Pollo, A. How Placebos Change the Patient's Brain. *Neuropsychopharmacol* 36, 339–354 (2011). https://doi.org/10.1038/npp.2010.81.

7 Michigan Parkinson Foundation. "Placebo effect and the treatment of Parkinson's disease," MPF website. Available at: https://parkinsonsmi.org/treatment/entry/placebo-effect-and-the-treatment-of-parkinsons-disease. (Accessed: 21 Jan. 2023.)

8   Fink J.S., The Placebo Effect in Clinical Trials in Parkinson's Disease. American Parkinson's Disease Association, https://www.apdaparkinson. org/article/the-placebo-effect-in-clinical-trials-in-parkinsons-disease/.

9   Hansen, B. J., Meyhoff, H. H., Nordling, J., Mensink, H. J., Mogensen, P., & Larsen, E. H. (1996). Placebo effects in the pharmacological treatment of uncomplicated benign prostatic hyperplasia. The ALFECH Study Group. *Scandinavian journal of urology and nephrology*, 30(5), 373–377. https://doi.org/10.3109/00365599609181313.

10   Kennedy, W. P. (1961). "The Nocebo Reaction," *Medical World*, Vol. 95 (September), p. 204. Available at: OMICS International, https://pubmed. ncbi.nlm.nih.gov/13752532/ (Accessed: 21 Jan. 2023.)

11   Ikemi, Y. and Nakagawa, S. (1962), "A psychosomatic study of contagious dermatitis," *Kyoshu Journal of Medical Science*, Vol. 13, pp. 335–350. https:// www.semanticscholar.org/paper/A-psychosomatic-study-of-contagious-dermatitis-Ikemi-Nakagawa/65442ac9d4e7a800a55734c65601d591957a 39a9.

12   Blasini, M. *et al.* (2018). "The Role of Patient-Practitioner Relationships in Placebo and Nocebo Phenomena," *Int Rev Neurobiol.*, January, 139, pp. 211–231. Available at: doi: 10.1016/bs.irn.2018.07.033. PMID: 30146048; PMCID: PMC6176716.

13   Park, L., Covi, U., Reprinted from the Archives of General Psychiatry April 1965, Vol. 12, pp. 336–345 Copyright 1965, by American Medical Association Nonblind Placebo Trial An Exploration of Neurotic Patients' Responses to Placebo When Its Inert Content Is Disclosed. https://www.researchgate. net/profile/Lee-Park-4/publication/9326576_Nonblind_placebo_trial_ An_exploration_of_neurotic_patients'_responses_to_placebo_when_ its_inret_content_is_disclosed/links/5a0b7e44a6fdccc69eda314f/ Nonblind-placebo-trial-An-exploration-of-neurotic-patients-responses-to-placebo-when-its-inret-content-is-disclosed.pdf

14   Kaptchuk, T. J. *et al.* (2010). "Placebos without Deception: A Randomized Controlled Trial in Irritable Bowel Syndrome," PLOS website, 22 December. Available at doi.org/10.1371/journal.pone.0015591 (Accessed: 21 Jan. 2023.)

15   Jacome, D. E. (2001). Transitional Interpersonality Thunderclap Headache. Headache: The Journal of Head and Face Pain, 41(3), 317–320. https:// doi.org/10.1046/j.1526-4610.2001.111006317.x.

16   Science Clarified, "Multiple Personality Disorder," Science Clarified website. Available at: www.scienceclarified.com/Ma-Mu/Multiple-Personality-Disorder.html (Accessed: 21 Jan. 2023.)

17 Waldvogel, B., Ullrich, A. and Strasburger, H. (2007). "Blind und sehend in einer person: schlussfolgerungen zur psychoneurobiologie des sehens" [Sighted and blind in one person: a case report and conclusions on the psychoneurobiology of vision], Nervenarzt, November, 78(11), pp.1303–9. German. Available at: doi: 10.1007/s00115-007-2309-x. PMID: 17611729. See also: https://pubmed.ncbi.nlm.nih.gov/17611729/ (Accessed: 21 Jan. 2023.)

18 Strasburger H, Waldvogel B. Sight and blindness in the same person: Gating in the visual system. Psych J. 2015 Dec;4(4):178–85. doi: 10.1002/pchj.109. Epub 2015 Oct 15. PMID: 26468893.

19 Cleveland Clinic, "Phantom Limb Pain," Cleveland Clinic website. Available at: https://my.clevelandclinic.org/health/diseases/12092-phantom-limb-pain (Accessed: 21 Jan. 2023.)

20 See "spontaneous remission."(n.d.). *Farlex Partner Medical Dictionary* (2012). Available at: https://medical-dictionary.thefreedictionary.com/spontaneous+remission (Accessed: 20 May, 2022.)

21 O'Regan B., Hirshberg C., *Spontaneous Remission: An Annotated Bibliography*, ISBN-13. 978-0943951171; Edition. 1st; Publisher. *Inst of Noetic Sciences*, Publication date. January 1, 1995.

CHAPTER 3

1 Epigraph: Sankey, J., Zen and the Art of Stand-up Comedy. Taylor & Francis 1998. ISBS.9780878300747.

2 Cleveland Clinic. Health Essentials. Skin. Oct. 2021. https://my.clevelandclinic.org/health/articles/10978-skin.

3 Milo, R. (2021). "Mapping cellular turnover sheds light on the balance between renewal and stability in our bodies," Weizmann Wonder Wander website, 15 February. Available at: https://wis-wander.weizmann.ac.il/life-sciences/cell-replacement-numbers (Accessed: 21 Jan. 2023.)

4 Manolagas S., Birth and Death of Bone Cells: Basic Regulatory Mechanisms and Implications for the Pathogenesis and Treatment of Osteoporosis, *Endocrine Reviews*, Volume 21, Issue 2, 1 April 2000, Pages 115–137, https://doi.org/10.1210/edrv.21.2.0395.

5 Office of the Surgeon General (US). Bone Health and Osteoporosis: A Report of the Surgeon General. Rockville (MD): Office of the Surgeon General (US); 2004. 2, The Basics of Bone in Health and Disease. Available from: https://www.ncbi.nlm.nih.gov/books/NBK45504/

6 Danese, E., Lippi, G., Sanchis-Gomar, F., Brocco, G., Rizzo, M., Banach, M., & Montagnana, M. (2017). Physical Exercise and DNA Injury:

Good or Evil? *Advances in clinical chemistry*, *81*, 193–230. https://doi. org/10.1016/bs.acc.2017.01.005.

7   *Time* Magazine: Science. The Fleeting Flesh. 1954. http://content.time. com/time/subscriber/article/0,33009,936455,00.html.

8   Benfatto, M., Pace, E., Davoli, I., Lucci, M., Francini, R., De Matteis, F., Scordo, A., Clozza, A., Grandi, M., Curceanu, C., Grigolini, P., Biophotons – new experimental data and analysis. May 01, 2023. Physics - Biological Physics; Quantitative Biology – Quantitative ©The SAO/NASA Astrophysics Data System. The ADS is operated by the Smithsonian Astrophysical Observatory Under NASA Cooperative Agreement. https://ui.adsabs.harvard.edu/abs/2023arXiv230509524B.

9   Popp, Fritz-Albert, Gu, Qiao, G. Li, Ke-Hsueh. Biophoton Emission: Experimental Background and Theoretical Approaches. ©The SAO/ NASA Astrophysics Data System. The ADS is operated by the Smithsonian Astrophysical Observatory Under NASA Cooperative Agreement.   https://ui.adsabs.harvard.edu/abs/1994MPLB....8.1269P/ abstract

10 Nomination Archive. NobelPrize.org. Nobel Prize Outreach AB 2023. Sun. 17 Sep 2023. https://www.nobelprize.org/nomination/archive/ show_people.php?id=3725.

11 Technically Gurwitsch was awarded the State Stalin Prize in 1941, however the Stalin award was renamed in 1957 and is now most known as the "USSR State Prize". "Gurwitsch (Gurvich), Alexander Gavrilovich." Encyclopaedia Judaica. Encyclopedia.com. (September 18, 2023). https:// www.encyclopedia.com/religion/encyclopedias-almanacs-transcripts- and-maps/gurwitsch-gurvich-alexander-gavrilovich

12 Gurwitsch L. D., Salkind S. (1929). Das mitogenetische verhalten des bluts carcinomatoser. Biochem. Z 211, 362.

13 Pesochensky B. S. (1947). Quenching of mitogenetic radiation of blood in cancer and precancerous diseases, in Collected Volume on Mitogenesis and the Theory of Biological Field (Moscow: Pub.house of the USSR Academy of Medical Sciences;), 102–114.

14 Gurwitsch A. G. (1923). Die natur des spezifischen erregers der zellteilung. Arch. Mikrosk. Anat. Und. Entw. Mech. 100, 11–40.

15 Gurwitsch A. G. (1924). Physicalisches uber mitogenetische strahlen. Arch. Mikrosk. Anat. Und. Entw. Mech. 103, 490–498.

16 N. Yang N., S.D. Ray, S.D., Krafts K., Cell Proliferation, 2014, Pages 761–765, ISBN 9780123864550. https://doi.org/10.1016/B978-0-12- 386454-3.00274-8.

17   Ackerman S. Discovering the Brain. Washington (DC): National Academies Press (US); 1992. 6, The Development and Shaping of the Brain. Available from: https://www.ncbi.nlm.nih.gov/books/NBK234146/

18   Kan, A., & Hodgkin, P. D. (2014). Mechanisms of cell division as regulators of acute immune response. Systems and synthetic biology, 8(3), 215–221. https://doi.org/10.1007/s11693-014-9149-3

19   Li, G., White, G., Connolly, C. and Marsh, D. (2002), Cell Proliferation and Apoptosis During Fracture Healing. J Bone Miner Res, 17: 791-799. https://doi.org/10.1359/jbmr.2002.17.5.791

20   Landén, N. X., Li, D., & Ståhle, M. (2016). Transition from inflammation to proliferation: a critical step during wound healing. Cellular and molecular life sciences: CMLS, 73(20), 3861–3885. https://doi.org/10.1007/s00018-016-2268-0

21   Sporn, M. B., & Harris, E. D. (1981). Proliferative Diseases. The American Journal of Medicine, 70(6), 1231–1236. https://doi.org/10.1016/0002-9343(81)90832-9.

22   Ponchel, F., Morgan, A. W., Bingham, S. J., Quinn, M., Buch, M., Verburg, R. J., Henwood, J., Douglas, S. H., Masurel, A., Conaghan, P., Gesinde, M., Taylor, J., Markham, A. F., Emery, P., van Laar, J. M., & Isaacs, J. D. (2002b). Dysregulated lymphocyte proliferation and differentiation in patients with rheumatoid arthritis. Blood, 100(13), 4550–4556. https://doi.org/10.1182/blood-2002-03-0671.

23   Cooper GM. The Cell: A Molecular Approach. 2nd edition. Sunderland (MA): Sinauer Associates; 2000. The Development and Causes of Cancer. Available from: https://www.ncbi.nlm.nih.gov/books/NBK9963/.

24   Varner, C., Dixon, L., & Simons, M. C. (2021). The Past, Present, and Future: A Discussion of Cadaver Use in Medical and Veterinary Education. Frontiers in veterinary science, 8, 720740. https://doi.org/10.3389/fvets.2021.720740.

25   Jeanette Der Bedrosian. Johns Hopkins Magazine. Winter 2016 Issue. https://hub.jhu.edu/magazine/2016/winter/cadavers-anatomy-medical-school/ (Accessed: 13 Feb. 2023.)

26   Popp, F. A., Li, K. H., Mei, W. P., Galle, M., & Neurohr, R. (1988). Physical aspects of biophotons. Experientia, 44(7), 576–585. https://doi.org/10.1007/bf01953305.

27   Sanders C. L. (2014). Speculations about Bystander and Biophotons. Dose-response: a publication of International Hormesis Society, 12(4), 515–517. https://doi.org/10.2203/dose-response.14-002.Sanders.

28 Chang, J. J., & Popp, F. A. (1998). Biological Organization: A Possible Mechanism Based on the Coherence of "Biophotons." Biophotons, 217–227. https://doi.org/10.1007/978-94-017-0928-6_16.

29 Y., Ma, J., ; Guo, Z.,Coherent properties of ultraweak photon emission from biological system and its application in medicine. Biophotonics Instrumentation and Analysis. 2001, Chiou, A., Podbielska, H.,Jacques, S.,V.4597. Oct,2001. p.36–42.doi.10.1117/12.446657.https://ui.adsabs.harvard.edu/abs/2001SPIE.4597...36Z. Provided by the SAO/NASA Astrophysics Data System. The ADS is operated by the Smithsonian Astrophysical Observatory Under NASA Cooperative Agreement.

30 Ives, J. A., van Wijk, E. P., Bat, N., Crawford, C., Walter, A., Jonas, W. B., van Wijk, R., & van der Greef, J. (2014). Ultraweak photon emission as a non-invasive health assessment: a systematic review. PloS one, 9(2), e87401. https://doi.org/10.1371/journal.pone.0087401

31 Science. Gov "Your Gateway to U.S. Federal Science https://www.science.gov/topicpages/u/ultraweak+photon+emission

32 Wijk RV, Wijk EP. An introduction to human biophoton emission. Forsch Komplementarmed Klass Naturheilkd. 2005 Apr;12(2):77–83. doi: 10.1159/000083763. PMID: 15947465.

33 Niggli, H. J., Tudisco, S., Privitera, G., Applegate, L. A., Scordino, A., & Musumeci, F. (2005). Laser-ultraviolet-A-induced ultraweak photon emission in mammalian cells. Journal of biomedical optics, 10(2), 024006. https://doi.org/10.1117/1.1899185

34 Park, S. H., Kim, J., & Koo, T. H. (2009). Magneto-acupuncture stimuli effects on ultraweak photon emission from hands of healthy persons. Journal of acupuncture and meridian studies, 2(1), 40–48. https://doi.org/10.1016/S2005-2901(09)60014-5

35 Emerging Technology from the arXiv. MIT Technology Review. "The Puzzling Role of Biophotons in the Brain." Dec. 17, 2010. https://www.technologyreview.com/2010/12/17/198375/the-puzzling-role-of-biophotons-in-the-brain/

36 Ibid. 28

37 Sun, Y., Wang, C., & Dai, J. (2010). Biophotons as neural communication signals demonstrated by in situ biophoton autography. Photochemical & photobiological sciences: Official journal of the European Photochemistry Association and the European Society for Photobiology, 9(3), 315–322. https://doi.org/10.1039/b9pp00125e.

38 Fels, D. (2009, April 1). Cellular Communication through Light. PLOS ONE. https://doi.org/10.1371/journal.pone.0005086.

39 Mitrofanis, J., Moro, C., Liebert, A., Hamilton, C., Pasqual, N., Jeffery, G., & Stone, J. (2022). The code of light: do neurons generate light to communicate and repair? Neural Regeneration Research, 17(6), 1251. https://doi.org/10.4103/1673-5374.327332.

40 Tang, R., & Dai, J. (2014). Biophoton signal transmission and processing in the brain. Journal of Photochemistry and Photobiology B: Biology, 139, 71–75. https://doi.org/10.1016/j.jphotobiol.2013.12.008.

41 Mayburov, S.N., (2009) "Coherent and Noncoherent Photonic Communications in Biological Systems," https://arxiv.org/pdf/0909.2676.pdf.

42 Dotta, B.T., Murugan, N.J., Karbowski, L.M. *et al.* Shifting wavelengths of ultraweak photon emissions from dying melanoma cells: their chemical enhancement and blocking are predicted by Cosic's theory of resonant recognition model for macromolecules. *Naturwissenschaften* 101, 87–94 (2014). https://doi.org/10.1007/s00114-013-1133-3

43 MIT Technology Review. Biophoton Communication. Can Cells Talk Using Light. May 2012. https://www.technologyreview.com/2012/05/22/185994/biophoton-communication-can-cells-talk-using-light/

44 Beloussov, L.V. and Baskakov, I.V. (1995) "A reproduction of the mitogenetic experiments of the Ourwitsch school on frog and fish cleaving eggs," in: L.V. Beloussov and F..A. Popp (eds.), Biophotonics, Bioinform Service, Moscow, pp. 447–456

45 Staxén, I., Bergounioux, C. & Bornman, J.F. "Effect of ultraviolet radiation on cell division and microtubule organization in Petunia hybrida protoplasts." Protoplasma 173, 70–76 (1993).

46 Ibid. 43

47 Ibid. 38

48 Hamouda, S. Khalifa, N., Belhasan, M., "Bio-Photon Research and Its Applications: A Review." International Journal of Interdisciplinary Research and Innovations. ISSN 2348-1226 (online) Vol. 6, Issue 1, pp: (35–46), Month: January–March 2018, https://www.researchgate.net/publication/343738204_Bio-Photon_Research_and_Its_Applications_A_Review.

49 Wang, Z., Wang, N., Li, Z., Xiao, F., Dai, J., Human high intelligence is involved in spectral redshift of biophotonic activities in the brain. Proceedings of the National Academy of Science. 2016, Aug., vol.113.,

p.8753–8758, doi.10.1073/pnas.1604855113. https://ui.adsabs.harvard. edu/abs/2016PNAS..113.8753W. Provided by the SAO/NASA Astrophysics Data System. The ADS is operated by the Smithsonian Astrophysical Observatory Under NASA Cooperative Agreement.

50 Ibid. 40

51 Rahnama, M., Tuszynski, J. A., Bokkon, I., Cifra, M., Sardar, P., Salari, V., (2011). "Emission of Biophotons and Neural Activity of the Brain." Journal of Integrative Neuroscience, 10(01), 65–88 https://doi. org/10.1142/S0219635211002622

52 Van Wijk, R., Bosman, S., Ackerman, J., & Wijk, E. V. (2008). Correlation between Fluctuations in Human Ultra-weak Photon Emission and EEG Alpha Rhythm. NeuroQuantology, 6(4). https://doi.org/10.14704/ nq.2008.6.4.201

53 Takeda M, Kobayashi M, Takayama M, Suzuki S, Ishida T, Ohnuki K, Moriya T, Ohuchi N. Biophoton detection as a novel technique for cancer imaging. Cancer Sci. 2004 Aug;95(8):656–61. doi: 10.1111/j.1349-7006.2004.tb03325.x. PMID: 15298728. https:// pubmed.ncbi.nlm.nih.gov/15298728/.

54 Murugan, N. J., Rouleau, N., Karbowski, L. M., & Persinger, M. A. (2018). Biophotonic markers of malignancy: Discriminating cancers using wavelength-specific biophotons. Biochemistry and Biophysics Reports, 13, 7–11. https://doi.org/10.1016/j.bbrep.2017.11.001.

55 Ibid. 53

56 Yang, M., Ding, W., Liu, Y., Fan, H., Bajpai, R. P., Fu, J., Pang, J., Zhao, X., & Han, J. (2017). Ultra-weak photon emission in healthy subjects and patients with type 2 diabetes: evidence for a non-invasive diagnostic tool. Photochemical &Amp; Photobiological Sciences, 16(5), 736–743. https://doi.org/10.1039/c6pp00431h.

57 Ibid.

58 Cifra, M., Brouder, C., Nerudová, M., Kučera, O., Biophotons, coherence and photocount statistics: A critical review. Journal of Luminescence, vol. 164, pp. 38–51 The SAO/NASA Astrophysics Data System. The ADS is operated by the Smithsonian Astrophysical Observatory Under NASA Cooperative Agreement. https://ui.adsabs.harvard.edu/ abs/2015JLum..164...38C/abstract.

59 Mayburov, S.N., "Coherent and Noncoherent Photonic Communications in Biological Systems," https://arxiv.org/abs/0909.2676.

60 Ibid. 39

61 Srinivasan, T. M. (2017). Biophotons as Subtle Energy Carriers. *International journal of yoga*, 10(2), 57–58. https://www.ncbi.nlm.nih.gov/pmc/articles/PMC5433113/

62 F.A.Popp and J.J.Chang discuss the informational character of biophotons, the role for biochemical reactivity as well as for growth regulation and spatio-temporal organization in living systems. https://link.springer.com/book/10.1007/978-94-017-0928-6.

63 Ibid. 51

64 Hamouda, Samir. (2020). Bio-Photon Research and Its Applications: A Review. 35–46.

65 Ibid. 37

66 Ibid. 40

67 Salari, V., Valian, H., Bassereh, H., Bókkon, I., & Barkhordari, A. (2015). Ultraweak photon emission in the brain. *Journal of integrative neuroscience*, 14(3), 419–429. https://doi.org/10.1142/S0219635215300012

CHAPTER 4

1 Epigraph: Supermundane.1938. Angi Yoga Society, Inc., New York https://agniyoga.org/ay_en/Supermundane.php

2 Isojima Y, Isoshima T, Nagai K, Kikuchi K, Nakagawa H, "Ultraweak biochemiluminescence detected from rat hippocampal slices," Neuroreport 6:658–660, 1995. https://pubmed.ncbi.nlm.nih.gov/7605921/.

3 Kobayashi M, Takeda M, Sato T, Yamazaki Y, Kaneko K, Ito K, Kato H, Inaba H, "Invivo imaging of spontaneous ultraweak photon emission from a rat's brain correlated with cerebral energy metabolism and oxidative stress," Neurosci Res 34:103–113, 1999.

4 Ibid. Chapter 3, 49

5 Salari, V., Rodrigues, S., Saglamyurek, E., ; Simon, C., Oblak, D., Are Brain-Computer Interfaces Feasible with Integrated Photonic Chips? November 01, 2021. Quantitative Biology - Neurons and Cognition; Physics – Biological. Physics; Physics - Medical Physics; Physics - Optics; Quantum Physics. The SAO/NASA Astrophysics Data System. The ADS is operated by the Smithsonian Astrophysical Observatory Under NASA Cooperative Agreement. https://ui.adsabs.harvard.edu/abs/2021arXiv211201249S

6 Zarkeshian, P., Kergan, T., Ghobadi, R., Nicola, W., Simon, C. Photons guided by axons may enable backpropagation-based learning in the brain. Scientific Reports. 2022.Dec. vol.12., p.20720. doi.10.1038/s41598-022-24871-6.https://ui.adsabs.harvard.edu/abs/2022NatSR..1220720Z,

Provided by the SAO/NASA Astrophysics Data System. The ADS is operated by the Smithsonian Astrophysical Observatory Under NASA Cooperative Agreement.

7   Van Wijk, E. P., Koch, H., Bosman, S., & Wijk, R. V. (2006). Anatomic Characterization of Human Ultra-Weak Photon Emission in Practitioners of Transcendental Meditation™ and Control Subjects. The Journal of Alternative and Complementary Medicine, 12(1), 31–38. https://doi.org/10.1089/acm.2006.12.31.

8   Van Wijk EP, Ackerman J, Van Wijk R. Effect of meditation on ultraweak photon emission from hands and forehead. Forsch Komplementarmed Klass Naturheilkd. 2005;12:107–12.

9   Van Wijk, E. P., Lüdtke, R., & Van Wijk, R. (2008). Differential effects of relaxation techniques on ultraweak photon emission. Journal of Alternative and Complementary Medicine (New York, N.Y.), 14(3), 241–250. https://doi.org/10.1089/acm.2007.7185

10 Van Wijk, E. P., Van Wijk, R., & Bajpai, R. P. (2008). Quantum squeezed state analysis of spontaneous ultra-weak light photon emission of practitioners of meditation and control subjects. Indian Journal of Experimental Biology, 46(5), 345–352.

11 Dotta, B. T., & Persinger, M. A. (2011). Increased Photon Emissions from the Right But Not the Left Hemisphere While Imagining White Light in the Dark: The Potential Connection Between Consciousness and Cerebral Light. Journal of Consciousness Exploration & Research, 2(10). http://jcer.com/index.php/jcj/article/view/190/203.

12 Zapata, F., Pastor-Ruiz, V., Ortega-Ojeda, F., Montalvo, G., & García-Ruiz, C. (2021). Increment of spontaneous human biophoton emission caused by anger emotional states. Proof of concept. Microchemical Journal, 169, 106558. https://doi.org/10.1016/j.microc.2021.106558.

13 Thornton, L. M., & Andersen, B. L. (2006). Psychoneuroimmunology examined: The role of subjective stress. Cellscience. https://pubmed.ncbi.nlm.nih.gov/18633462/

14 Scanlan, J. M., Vitaliano, P. P., Zhang, J., Savage, M., & Ochs, H. D. (2001). Lymphocyte proliferation is associated with gender, caregiving, and psychosocial variables in older adults. Journal of Behavioral Medicine, 24(6), 537–559. https://doi.org/10.1023/a:1012987226388.

15 Dai, S., Mo, Y., Wang, Y., Xiang, B., Liao, Q., Zhou, M., Li, X., Li, Y., Xiong, W., Li, G., Guo, C., & Zeng, Z. (2020). Chronic Stress Promotes Cancer Development. Frontiers in Oncology, 10, 1492. https://doi.org/10.3389/fonc.2020.01492.

16 Vignjević Petrinović S., Milošević M. S., Marković D., Momčilović S., Interplay between stress and cancer—A focus on inflammation. Frontiers in Physiology. V.14. 2023. https://www.frontiersin.org/articles/10.3389/fphys.2023.1119095. DOI.10.3389/fphys.2023.1119095

17 Yegorov, Y. E., Poznyak, A. V., Nikiforov, N. G., Sobenin, I. A., & Orekhov, A. N. (2020). The Link between Chronic Stress and Accelerated Aging. *Biomedicines, 8*(7), 198. https://doi.org/10.3390/biomedicines8070198

18 Chen, Y., & Lyga, J. (2014). Brain-skin connection: stress, inflammation and skin aging. Inflammation & allergy drug targets, 13(3), 177–190. https://doi.org/10.2174/1871528113666140522104422.

19 Gouin, J. P., Kiecolt-Glaser, J. K., Malarkey, W. B., & Glaser, R. (2008). The influence of anger expression on wound healing. Brain, Behavior, and Immunity, 22(5), 699–708. https://doi.org/10.1016/j.bbi.2007.10.013

20 Kiecolt-Glaser JK, Page GG, Marucha PT, et al. Psychological influences on surgical recovery: Perspectives from psychoneuroimmunology. *Am Psychol.* 1998;53:1209–18.

21 Rosenberger, P. H., Jokl, P., & Ickovics, J. (2006). Psychosocial factors and surgical outcomes: an evidence-based literature review. *The Journal of the American Academy of Orthopaedic Surgeons, 14*(7), 397–405. https://doi.org/10.5435/00124635-200607000-00002.

22 Ronaldson, A., Poole, L., Kidd, T., Leigh, E., Jahangiri, M., & Steptoe, A. (2014). Optimism measured pre-operatively is associated with reduced pain intensity and physical symptom reporting after coronary artery bypass graft surgery. Journal of Psychosomatic Research, 77(4), 278–282. https://doi.org/10.1016/j.jpsychores.2014.07.018.

23 Kubzansky, L. D., & Thurston, R. C. (2007). Emotional Vitality and Incident Coronary Heart Disease. Archives of General Psychiatry, 64(12), 1393. https://doi.org/10.1001/archpsyc.64.12.1393

24 Lee, L. O., James, P., Zevon, E. S., Kim, E. S., Trudel-Fitzgerald, C., Spiro, A., Grodstein, F., & Kubzansky, L. D. (2019). Optimism is associated with exceptional longevity in 2 epidemiologic cohorts of men and women. Proceedings of the National Academy of Sciences, 116(37), 18357–18362. https://doi.org/10.1073/pnas.1900712116.

25 Koga, H. K., Trudel-Fitzgerald, C., Lee, L. O., James, P., Kroenke, C., Garcia, L., Shadyab, A. H., Salmoirago-Blotcher, E., Manson, J. E., Grodstein, F., & Kubzansky, L. D. (2022). Optimism, lifestyle, and longevity in a racially diverse cohort of women. Journal of the American

Geriatrics Society, 70(10), 2793–2804. https://doi.org/10.1111/jgs.17897.

26 Wilhelm, M., Winkler, A., Rief, W., & Doering, B. K. (2016). Effect of placebo groups on blood pressure in hypertension: a meta-analysis of beta-blocker trials. *Journal of the American Society of Hypertension: JASH*, 10(12), 917–929. https://doi.org/10.1016/j.jash.2016.10.009.

27 McGlashan, T. M., Evans, F. J., and Orne, M. T. The nature of hypnotic analgesia and placebo response to experimental pain. Psychosomatic Medicine, 1969, 31, 227–246, https://www.psych.upenn.edu/history/orne/mcglashanetal1969psychosommed227244.html.

28 Ibid. Chapter 2, 12

29 Scott, D.J., Stohler, C.S., Egnatuk, C.M., Wang, H., Koeppe, R.A., Zubieta, J.K. Individual differences in reward responding explain placebo-induced expectations and effects Neuron, 55 (2007), pp. 325–336 https://doi.org/10.1016/j.neuron.2007.06.028.

30 Ibid. Chapter 3, 51

31 F.A.Popp and J.J.Chang discuss the informational character of biophotons, the role for biochemical reactivity as well as for growth regulation and spatio-temporal organization in living systems. https://link.springer.com/book/10.1007/978-94-017-0928-6.

32 Hopper, Annedore & Ciorciari, Joseph & Johnson, Gillian & Spensley, John & Sergejew, Alex & Stough, Con. (2002). EEG Coherence and Dissociative Identity Disorder. Journal of Trauma & Dissociation - J TRAUMA DISSOCIATION. 3. 75-88. 10.1300/J229v03n01_06.

33 Srivastava, K. K., & Kumar, R. (2015). Stress, oxidative injury and disease. Indian journal of clinical biochemistry: IJCB, 30(1), 3–10. https://doi.org/10.1007/s12291-014-0441-5. https://www.ncbi.nlm.nih.gov/pmc/articles/PMC4310835/.

34 Kobayashi K, Okabe H, Kawano S, Hidaka Y, Hara K. Biophoton emission induced by heat shock. PLoS One. 2014 Aug 25;9(8):e105700. doi: 10.1371/journal.pone.0105700. PMID: 25153902; PMCID: PMC4143285.

35 Kobayashi M., Takeda M., Sato T., Yamazaki Y., Kaneko K., Ito K., Kato H., Inaba H. In vivo imaging of spontaneous ultraweak photon emission from a rat's brain correlated with cerebral energy metabolism and oxidative stress. Neurosci Res. 1999 Jul;34(2):103–13. doi: 10.1016/s0168-0102(99)00040-1. PMID: 10498336.

36 Winkler R., Guttenberger H., Klima H. Ultraweak and induced photon emission after wounding of plants. Photochem Photobiol. 2009 Jul-Aug;85(4):962–5. doi: 10.1111/j.1751-1097.2009.00537.x. Epub 2009 Feb 23. PMID: 19254235.

37 Fedoroff N., Redox regulatory mechanisms in cellular stress responses. Ann Bot. 2006 Aug;98(2):289–300. doi: 10.1093/aob/mcl128. Epub 2006 Jun 21. PMID: 16790465; PMCID: PMC2803466.

38 Ibid. Chapter 3, 51

39 Bókkon, I., Salari, V., Tuszynski, J., & Antal, I. (2010). Estimation of the number of biophotons involved in the visual perception of a single-object image: Biophoton intensity can be considerably higher inside cells than outside. Journal of Photochemistry and Photobiology B: Biology, 100(3), 160–166. https://doi.org/10.1016/j.jphotobiol.2010.06.001.

40 Du, J., Deng, T., Cao, B., Wang, Z., Yang, M., & Han, J. (2023). The application and trend of ultra-weak photon emission in biology and medicine. Frontiers in chemistry, 11, 1140128. https://doi.org/10.3389/fchem.2023.1140128

41 Kent, J. B., Jin, L., & Li, X. J. (2020). Quantifying Biofield Therapy through Biophoton Emission in a Cellular Model. Journal of scientific exploration 34(3), 434–454. https://doi.org/10.31275/20201691

42 Cleveland Clinic. Health Essentials. https://health.clevelandclinic.org/reiki/ What Is Reiki, and Does it Really Work? Aug. 30, 2021.

43 ThinkTree. St George's Hospital. https://thinktreehub.com/st-georges-hospital-and-reiki/

44 Ross, C., Blau M., Sheridan K., STAT News. Medicine with a side of mysticism: Top hospitals promote unproven therapies. March 7, 2017. https://www.statnews.com/2017/03/07/alternative-medicine-hospitals-promote/

45 Ibid. Chapter 3, 39

46 Kara, C., Selamet, H., Gökmenoğlu, C., & Kara, N. (2018). Low level laser therapy induces increased viability and proliferation in isolated cancer cells. Cell proliferation, 51(2), e12417. https://doi.org/10.1111/cpr.12417.

47 Lin, Yi-Yuan, Shin-Yi Lee, and Yu-Jung Cheng. 2023. "Low-Level Laser Therapy Induces Melanoma Tumor Growth by Promoting Angiogenesis" Life 13, no. 2: 320. https://doi.org/10.3390/life13020320

CHAPTER 5

1 Epigraph: Albert Einstein, William Hermanns, in: Einstein and the Poet: In Search of the Cosmic Man, Branden Books, 1 April 1983.

2 Canlon B., Theorell T., Hasson D., Associations between stress and hearing problems in humans, Hearing Research, Volume 295,2013, Pages 9–15, ISSN 0378-5955, https://doi.org/10.1016/j.heares.2012.08.015.

3 Sabel, B.A., Wang, J., Cárdenas-Morales, L. *et al.* Mental stress as consequence and cause of vision loss: the dawn of psychosomatic ophthalmology for preventive and personalized medicine. *EPMA Journal* 9, 133–160 (2018). https://doi.org/10.1007/s13167-018-0136-8.

4 Lisman, J., & Sternberg, E. J. (2013). Habit and nonhabit systems for unconscious and conscious behavior: implications for multitasking. *Journal of cognitive neuroscience, 25*(2), 273–283. https://doi.org/10.1162/jocn_a_00319

5 Bargh, J. A., & Morsella, E. (2008). The Unconscious Mind. *Perspectives on psychological science: a journal of the Association for Psychological Science, 3*(1), 73–79. https://doi.org/10.1111/j.1745-6916.2008.00064.x

6 Tryon, W. W. (2014). *Cognitive neuroscience and psychotherapy: Network Principles for a Unified Theory.* New York: Academic Press.

7 Baumann, K. (1999) "The Concept of Human Acts Revisited. St Thomas and the Unconscious in Freedom", in: Gregorianum 80 (1999) 147–171.

8 Westen, D. (1999). "The Scientific Status of Unconscious Processes: Is Freud Really Dead?," *Journal of the American Psychoanalytic Association,* Vol. 47(4):1061–1106. Available at: doi:10.1177/000306519904700404 (Accessed: 21 Jan. 2023.)

9 Bargh, J. A., & Morsella, E. (2008). The Unconscious Mind. *Perspectives on psychological science: a journal of the Association for Psychological Science, 3*(1), 73–79. https://doi.org/10.1111/j.1745–6916.2008.00064.x.

10 Bargh J. A. (2019). The modern unconscious. *World psychiatry: official journal of the World Psychiatric Association (WPA), 18*(2), 225–226. https://doi.org/10.1002/wps.20625 https://onlinelibrary.wiley.com/doi/10.1002/wps.20625.

11 Luodong Y., Haohao L., Yao M., Yan S., Anxin G., Guiqing Z., Chaomeng L. Dynamic changes in brain structure in patients with post-traumatic stress disorder after motor vehicle accident: A voxel-based morphometry-based follow-up study. Frontiers in Psychology. VOL.13. YEAR. 2022. https://www.frontiersin.org/articles/10.3389/fpsyg.2022.1018276. DOI=10.3389/fpsyg.2022.1018276

12 Chaney A, Carballedo A, Amico F, Fagan A, Skokauskas N, Meaney J, Frodl T. Effect of childhood maltreatment on brain structure in adult

patients with major depressive disorder and healthy participants. J Psychiatry Neurosci. 2014 Jan;39(1):50–9. doi: 10.1503/jpn.120208. PMID: 23900024; PMCID: PMC3868665.

13 Peverill, M., Rosen M., Lucy A. Lurie, Kelly A. Sambrook, Margaret A. Sheridan, Katie A. McLaughlin, Childhood trauma and brain structure in children and adolescents, Developmental Cognitive Neuroscience, Volume 59, 2023, 101180, ISSN 1878-9293.

14 Penfield, W., Boldrey, E., Somatic motor and sensory representation in the cerebral cortex of man as studied by electrical stimulation, *Brain*, Volume 60, Issue 4, December 1937, Pages 389–443, https://doi.org/10.1093/brain/60.4.389.

15 Photo Credit. Spencer Sutton/Science Source Images.

16 Kropf, E. et al. (2019). "From anatomy to function: the role of the somatosensory cortex in emotional regulation," *Braz J Psychiatry*, May-June, Vol. 41:3, pp.261–9. Available at: doi: 10.1590/1516-4446-2018-0183. Epub 6 December, 2018. PMID: 30540029; PMCID: PMC6794131. (Accessed: 21 Jan. 2023.)

17 Penfield, W., M. E. Faulk, Jr., "The Insula: Further Observations On Its Function." Brain, Volume 78, Issue 4, December 1955, Pages 445–470, doi.org/10.1093/brain/78.4.445

18 Fiol, M. E., Leppik, I. E., Mireles, R., & Maxwell, R. (1988). Ictus emeticus and the insular cortex. Epilepsy Research, 2(2), 127–131. https://doi.org/10.1016/0920-1211(88)90030-7

19 Ibid. Chapter 2, 15

20 Ibid. Chapter 3, 37

21 Kassam, K. S., Markey, A. R., Cherkassky, V. L., Loewenstein, G., & Just, M. A. (2013). Identifying Emotions on the Basis of Neural Activation. *PloS one*, 8(6), e66032. https://doi.org/10.1371/journal.pone.0066032

22 Ibid.

23 Rea, Shilo. Press Release: Carnegie Mellon Researchers Identify Emotions Based on Brain Activity.2013. https://www.cmu.edu/news/stories/archives/2013/june/june19_identifyingemotions.html

24 Uvnas-Moberg, K., & Petersson, M. (2005). Oxytocin, ein Vermittler von Antistress, Wohlbefinden, sozialer Interaktion, Wachstum und Heilung [Oxytocin, a mediator of anti-stress, well-being, social interaction, growth and healing]. Zeitschrift fur Psychosomatische Medizin und Psychotherapie, 51(1), 57–80. https://doi.org/10.13109/zptm.2005.51.1.57

25 Sumioka H, Nakae A, Kanai R, Ishiguro H. Huggable communication medium decreases cortisol levels. Sci Rep. 2013 Oct 23;3:3034. doi: 10.1038/srep03034. PMID: 24150186; PMCID: PMC3805974.

26 Bromberg-Martin ES, Matsumoto M, Hikosaka O. Dopamine in motivational control: rewarding, aversive, and alerting. Neuron. 2010 Dec 9;68(5):815–34. doi: 10.1016/j.neuron.2010.11.022. PMID: 21144997; PMCID: PMC3032992.

27 Hartston, H. The case for compulsive shopping as an addiction. J Psychoactive Drugs. 2012 Jan-Mar;44(1):64–7. doi:10.1080/02791072.2012.660110. PMID: 22641966.

28 Gepshtein, S., Li, X., Snider, J., Plank, M., Lee, D., & Poizner, H. (2014). Dopamine function and the efficiency of human movement. *Journal of cognitive neuroscience, 26*(3), 645–657. https://doi.org/10.1162/jocn_a_00503.

29 Ibid. 24

30 American Associations for Neurological Surgeons. Parkinson's Disease. https://www.aans.org/en/Patients/Neurosurgical-Conditions-and-Treatments/Parkinsons-Disease#:~:text=Studies%20have%20shown%20that%20symptoms,muscle%20cells%20involved%20in%20movement.

31 Feldman, C. H. et al. (2019). "Association of Childhood Abuse with Incident Systemic Lupus Erythematosus in Adulthood in a Longitudinal Cohort of Women," *J Rheumatol*, 46(12), pp.1589–1596. Available at: doi: 10.3899/jrheum.190009. Epub 15 May, 2019. PMID: 31092723; PMCID: PMC6856423. (Accessed: 21 Jan. 2023.)

32 Lupus Foundation of America. Childhood Abuse May Increase Risk of Lupus in Later Years. December. 2019. https://www.lupus.org/news/childhood-abuse-may-increase-risk-of-lupus-in-later-years (Accessed: 21 Jan. 2023.)

33 Hackett, R. A., Hudson, J. L. and Chilcot, J. (2020) "Loneliness and type 2 diabetes incidence: findings from the English Longitudinal Study of Ageing," *Diabetologia*, 15 September, Vol.63, pp. 2329–2338. Available at: https://doi.org/10.1007/s00125-020-05258-6. (Accessed: 21 Jan. 2023.)

34 Rabbing, L., Bjørkelo, B., Langvik, E., "Upper and lower musculoskeletal back pain, stress, physical activity, and organisational work support: An exploratory study of police investigative interviewers," Health Psychology Open, vol. 9, no. 2, 2022. doi.org/10.1177/20551029221146396.

35 Ibid. Chapter 2, 15

36 Dai, S., Mo, Y., Wang, Y., Xiang, B., Liao, Q., Zhou, M., Li, X., Li, Y., Xiong, W., Li, G., Guo, C., & Zeng, Z. (2020). Chronic Stress Promotes Cancer

Development. *Frontiers in oncology*, *10*, 1492. https://doi.org/10.3389/fonc.2020.01492

37 Chen, Y., & Lyga, J. (2014). Brain-skin connection: stress, inflammation and skin aging. Inflammation & allergy drug targets, 13(3), 177–190. https://doi.org/10.2174/1871528113666140522104422

38 Ibid. Chapter 4, 17

39 Gouin, J. P., Kiecolt-Glaser, J. K., Malarkey, W. B., & Glaser, R. (2008). The influence of anger expression on wound healing. Brain, Behavior, and Immunity, 22(5), 699–708. https://doi.org/10.1016/j.bbi.2007.10.013

40 Kiecolt-Glaser JK, Page GG, Marucha PT, et al. Psychological influences on surgical recovery: Perspectives from psychoneuroimmunology. *Am Psychol.* 1998;53:1209–18.

41 Ibid. Chapter 4, 22

42 Srivastava, K. K. and Kumar R. (2015). "Stress, oxidative injury and disease", Indian J Clin Biochem. 30(1), pp.3–10. Available at: doi: 10.1007/s12291-014-0441-5.

43 Cleveland Clinic. Can You Die of a Broken Heart? HealthEssentials Newsletter. Feb. 12,2020. https://health.clevelandclinic.org/can-die-broken-heart-emotional-questions/

44 Cleveland Clinic. It's True (But Rare) That You Can Be Scared to Death. HealthEssentials Newsletter. Oct. 12,2020. https://health.clevelandclinic.org/its-true-we-can-be-scared-to-death/

45 Shin, J. H., Lee, H. K., Choi, C. G., Suh, D. C., Kim, C. J., Hong, S. K., & Na, D. G. (2001). MR imaging of central diabetes insipidus: a pictorial essay. *Korean journal of radiology*, *2*(4), 222–230. https://doi.org/10.3348/kjr.2001.2.4.222

46 Ibid. Chapter 4, 24

47 Ibid. Chapter 4, 25

48 Ibid. Chapter 4, 22

CHAPTER 6

1 Epigraph: Gluck, L. (2022). The Wild Iris. United States: HarperCollins.

2 Freud S: Beyond the Pleasure Principle (1920), translated and edited by Strachey J. New York, WW Norton, 1961.

3 Merriam-Webster. (n.d.). Repetition compulsion. In Merriam-Webster.com medical dictionary. Retrieved February 8, 2023, from https://www.merriam-webster.com/medical/repetition%20compulsion.

4 Levy M. S. (1998). A helpful way to conceptualize and understand reenactments. *The Journal of psychotherapy practice and research*, 7(3), 227–235.

5 The American Psychological Association. Reenactment. Retrieved February 8, 2023, from https://dictionary.apa.org/reenactment.

6 Bibring, E. (1943). *"The Conception of the Repetition Compulsion"*. *The Psychoanalytic Quarterly*. 12 (4): 486–519. doi:10.1080/21674086.1943.11925548.

7 Walker, H. E., Freud, J. S., Ellis, R. A., Fraine, S. M., & Wilson, L. C. (2019). The Prevalence of Sexual Revictimization: A Meta-Analytic Review. *Trauma, Violence, & Abuse*, 20(1), 67–80. https://doi.org/10.1177/1524838017692364

8 Van der Kolk B. A. (1989). The compulsion to repeat the trauma. Re-enactment, revictimization, and masochism. *The Psychiatric clinics of North America*, 12(2), 389–411.

9 Office for National Statistics. https://www.ons.gov.uk/peoplepopulationandcommunity/crimeandjustice/articles/peoplewhowereabusedaschildrenaremorelikelytobeabusedasanadult/2017-09-27.

10 Erel, V. K., & Özkan, H. S. (2017). Thermal camera as a pain monitor. Journal of pain research, 10, 2827–2832. https://doi.org/10.2147/JPR.S151370

11 Lahiri BB, Bagavathiappan S, Jayakumar T, Philip J. Medical applications of infrared thermography: A review. Infrared Phys. Technol. 2012; 55(4):221-235. https://doi.org/10.1016/j.infrared.2012.03.007

12 Gillmore, B., Chevalier, G. and Kasian, S. (2023). Resolving Specific Psychological Stressors Can Instantly Reduce or Relieve Chronic Neck Pain and Upper Back Pain: Case Reports. Health, 15, 1116-1149. doi: 10.4236/health.2023.1510076.

CHAPTER 7

1 Epigraph: A maxim of Hill's, specifically cited as such, in *Success Through a Positive Mental Attitude* (1960), co-authored with W. Clement Stone, Ch. 14, p. 222.

2 Kirman, R. Psychology Today. Why Are We Blinded by Love? Here's what psychoanalysts say is the answer. Posted May 15, 2023

3 Bromberg (1994), "Speak! that I may see you": Some reflections on dissociation, reality, and psychoanalytic listening. In: Standing in the Spaces: Essays on Clinical Process, Trauma and Dissociation. Hillsdale, NJ: The Analytic Press, 1998

4 Swami V., Furnham A., The British Psychological Society. 18 February 2008. https://www.bps.org.uk/psychologist/love-really-so-blind. Accessed March 16, 2023

5   "The Origins of Attachment Theory: John Bowlby and Mary Ainsworth", *Developmental Psychology*, Vol.28, pp.759–75. Available at: www.psychology. sunysb.edu/attachment/online/inge_origins.pdf. For more on attachment theory, see also Fraley, R. C. "Adult Attachment Theory and Research". Available at: http://labs.psychology.illinois.edu/~rcfraley/attachment. htm.

6   Aurelius, M. (2002). *Meditations*. Random House.

7   Letter to Dr. H. L. Gordon (May 3, 1949 - AEA 58-217). Einstein and Michelson - the Context of Discovery and the Context of Justification. Stachel, J.,.Astronomische Nachrichten, Vol.303, Issue 1, p. 47, 1982. 1982AN....303...47Shttps://adsabs.harvard.edu/full/1982AN....303...47S.

8   Ibid. Chapter 5, 1. p16

9   Grau C, Ginhoux R, Riera A, Nguyen TL, Chauvat H, Berg M, et al. (2014) Conscious Brain-to-Brain Communication in Humans Using Non-Invasive Technologies. PLoS ONE 9(8): e105225. https://doi. org/10.1371/journal.pone.0105225

10 Scientists Prove That Telepathic Communication Is Within Reach https://www.smithsonianmag.com/innovation/scientists-prove-that-telepathic-communication-is-within-reach-180952868/

11 Puthoff, H. E. (n.d.). "CIA-Initiated Remote Viewing At Stanford Research Institute," Institute for Advanced Studies at Austin. Available at: www.newdualism.org/papers/H.Puthoff/CIA-Initiated%20Remote%20 Viewing%20At%20Stanford%20Research%20Institute.htm.

12 CNN.News Briefs. "Carter: CIA used psychic to help find missing plane". September 21, 1995. Web posted at 12:54 p.m. EDT. ATLANTA, Georgia (CNN). http://www.cnn.com/US/Newsbriefs/9509/9-21/am/ index.html.

CHAPTER 8

1   Epigraph: Albert Einstein, *Cosmic Religion: With Other Opinions and Aphorisms* (1931) by Albert Einstein, p. 97; also in *Transformation: Arts, Communication, Environment* (1950) by Harry Holtzman, p. 138.

2   Dijkstra, N., Fleming, S.M. Subjective signal strength distinguishes reality from imagination. *Nat Commun* 14, 1627 (2023). https://doi.org/10.1038/ s41467-023-37322-1

3   Pascual-Leone, A., Nguyet, D., Cohen, L. G., Brasil-Neto, J. P., Cammarota, A., & Hallett, M. (1995). Modulation of muscle responses evoked by transcranial magnetic stimulation during the acquisition of

new fine motor skills. *Journal of neurophysiology*, *74*(3), 1037–1045. https://doi.org/10.1152/jn.1995.74.3.1037.

4   University of Colorado at Boulder. "Your brain on imagination: It's a lot like reality, study shows." ScienceDaily. www.sciencedaily.com/releases/2018/12/181210144943.htm (accessed February 4, 2023).

CHAPTER 9

1   Epigraph: Browne, T., Sir, 1605-1682. Sir Thomas Browne's Religio Medici, Urn Burial, Christian Morals, and Other Essays. London: W. Scott, 1886.

2   Abel, E. L., & Kruger, M. L. (2010). Smile Intensity in Photographs Predicts Longevity. Psychological Science, 21(4), 542–544. https://doi.org/10.1177/0956797610363775.

3   Blood AJ, Zatorre RJ. Intensely pleasurable responses to music correlate with activity in brain regions implicated in reward and emotion. Proc Natl Acad Sci U S A. 2001 Sep 25;98(20):11818–23. doi: 10.1073/pnas.191355898. PMID: 11573015; PMCID: PMC58814.

4   Zatorre R. J. (2015). Musical pleasure and reward: mechanisms and dysfunction. *Annals of the New York Academy of Sciences, 1337*, 202–211. https://doi.org/10.1111/nyas.12677.

5   Ferreri, L., Mas-Herrero E.,Zatorre R.J.., Ripollés, P., Gomez-Andres A., Alicart H., Olivé, G., Marco-Pallarés, J., Antonijoan, R. M., Valle, M., Riba J., Rodriguez-Fornells, A., Dopamine modulates the reward experiences elicited by music. 2019. Proceedings of the National Academy of Sciences. P 3793-3798. V 116. N 9 doi:10.1073/pnas.1811878116.

6   Dunbar, R. I., Kaskatis, K., MacDonald, I., & Barra, V. (2012). Performance of music elevates pain threshold and positive affect: implications for the evolutionary function of music. *Evolutionary psychology: an international journal of evolutionary approaches to psychology and behavior, 10*(4), 688–702.

CHAPTER 10

1   Epigraph: Watts, A. (1966). *The book: On the taboo against knowing who you are.* Pantheon Books. P. 83

2   Santaularia, J., Johnson, M., Hart, L. *et al.* Relationships between sexual violence and chronic disease: a cross-sectional study. *BMC Public Health* 14, 1286 (2014). https://doi.org/10.1186/1471-2458-14-1286.

CHAPTER 11

1 Ibid. Chapter 5, 1. p137
2 Sabel, B.A., Wang, J., Cárdenas-Morales, L. et al. Mental stress as consequence and cause of vision loss: the dawn of psychosomatic ophthalmology for preventive and personalized medicine. EPMA Journal 9, 133–160 (2018). https://doi.org/10.1007/s13167-018-0136-8.
3 Birnbaum, M. H., & Thomann, K. (1996). Visual function in multiple personality disorder. Journal of the American Optometric Association, 67(6), 327–334.
4 Ibid. Chapter 2, 17
5 Ibid. Chapter 5, 35
6 Haendel, M., Vasilevsky, N., Unni, D., Bologa, C., Harris, N., Rehm, H., Hamosh, A., Baynam, G., Groza, T., McMurry, J., Dawkins, H., Rath, A., Thaxon, C., Bocci, G., Joachimiak, M. P., Köhler, S., Robinson, P. N., Mungall, C., & Oprea, T. I. (2020). How many rare diseases are there?. Nature reviews. Drug discovery, 19(2), 77–78. https://doi.org/10.1038/d41573-019-00180-y.
7 Golabchi, A., & Sarrafzadegan, N. (2011). Takotsubo cardiomyopathy or broken heart syndrome: A review article. *Journal of research in medical sciences: the official journal of Isfahan University of Medical Sciences, 16*(3), 340–345.

CHAPTER 12

1 Epigraph: Jung, C. *Modern Man in Search of a Soul* (1933). P. 69

CHAPTER 13

1 Epigraph: Mother Teresa. Interview by Edward W. Desmond in *TIME* magazine (4 December 1989)
2 Stanhope, R., Wilks, Z., & Hamill, G. (1994). Failure to grow: lack of food or lack of love?. Professional care of mother and child, 4(8), 234–237.
3 Doeker, B., Simić-Schleicher, Hauffa, B. P., & Andler, W. (1999). Psychosozialer Kleinwuchs maskiert als Wachstumshormonmangel [Psychosocially stunted growth masked as growth hormone deficiency]. Klinische Padiatrie, 211(5), 394–398. https://doi.org/10.1055/s-2008-1043818.
4 Burunat, E. (2016) Love Is Not an Emotion. Psychology, 7, 1883-1910. doi: 10.4236/psych.2016.714173.
5 Baars, Conrad W. *Doctor of the Heart.* Staten Island, NY: Alba House, 1996.
6 National Academies of Sciences, Engineering, and Medicine. 2020. Social Isolation and Loneliness in Older Adults: Opportunities for the Health

Care System. Washington, DC: The National Academies Press. https://doi.org/10.17226/25663.

7 Grannan,. "Can You Really Be Scared to Death?" *Encyclopedia Britannica*, October 1, 2016. https://www.britannica.com/story/can-you-really-be-scared-to-death.

8 Springer, K. W., Sheridan, J., Kuo, D., & Carnes, M. (2003). The long-term health outcomes of childhood abuse. An overview and a call to action. *Journal of general internal medicine*, *18*(10), 864–870. https://doi.org/10.1046/j.1525-1497.2003.20918.x.

9 Klonsky E. D. (2009). The functions of self-injury in young adults who cut themselves: clarifying the evidence for affect-regulation. *Psychiatry research*, *166*(2–3), 260–268. https://doi.org/10.1016/j.psychres.2008.02.008. https://www.ncbi.nlm.nih.gov/pmc/articles/PMC2723954/ (The appendix lists emotional experiences).

10 Peretti, Peter & Clark, Denise & Johnson, Pat. (1983). Affect of parental rejection on negative attention-seeking classroom behaviors. Indian journal of psychiatry. 25. 185–9.

11 Robison, J., Gallup."In Praise of Praising Your Employees. Frequent recognition is a surefire—and affordable—way to boost employee engagement." https://www.gallup.com/workplace/236951/praise-praising-employees.aspx

CHAPTER 14

1 Epigraph: Durant, W., *The Story of Philosophy* (1926), p. 76. The quoted phrases within the quotation are from the Nicomachean Ethics, Book II, 4; Book I, 7.

CHAPTER 15

1 Epigraph: Quotes reported in Josiah Hotchkiss Gilbert, *Dictionary of Burning Words of Brilliant Writers* (1895). P. 6

A Final Note

1 Centola, Damon & Becker, Joshua & Brackbill, Devon & Baronchelli, Andrea. (2018). Experimental evidence for tipping points in social convention. Science. 360. 1116-1119. 10.1126/science.aas8827.

2 Dall T., Reynolds R., Chakrabarti, R., Chylak, D., Jones, K., Iacobucci W., Association for Medical Colleges. "The Complexities of Physician Supply and Demand: Projections From 2019 to

2034." June 2021. https://www.aamc.org/media/54681/download
https://www.ama-assn.org/practice-management/sustainability/
doctor-shortages-are-here-and-they-ll-get-worse-if-we-don-t-act

3 The Health Foundation. A quarter of GP and general practice nursing
posts could be vacant in 10 years 25. July 2022 https://www.health.org.
uk/news-and-comment/news/a-quarter-of-gp-and-general-practice-
nursing-posts-could-be-vacant-in-10-years#:~:text=There%20is%20
currently%20a%20shortage,the%20rising%20need%20for%20care.

ACKNOWLEDGMENTS

1 Epigraph: Chapter 5, 1. p88

ACKNOWLEDGMENTS

I couldn't have come to my conclusions without the discoveries before me of great scientists.

—Albert Einstein[1]

As I type the final words of this book, my heart is overflowing. I love that you are here. I am filled with hope and anticipation for you and your journey of self-healing. I'm also excited for our future—that we can embrace a spirit-full awakening that will not only empower each individual person but also encourage a paradigm shift in our world that will benefit generations to come.

My heart is full of gratitude for all the support I have received on this journey. As the well-known proverb states, "It takes a village to raise a child." The same is true for birthing this book; it took a village of incredible people.

My first gratitude is always to the Universe, as none of this would be possible without the guidance and support that I receive on this level.

To my wonderful agents, Kristen Moeller and Bill Gladstone, thank you for all that you did and continue to do. I appreciate your expertise and support and for helping me bring this book into the world. I am grateful!

To Dr. Hillary Smith, I am so grateful to you. After my recovery, my biggest desire was to show people the power that our minds hold for healing, so they could see with their own eyes that we really can heal ourselves and release our own pain. It was you and your expertise in thermography that made that possible to demonstrate these results under live medical thermal imaging. Thank you!

To Gaetan Chevalier, thank you for being you, for your heart and for your kindness. Your role in helping with the study and working on publications for journals has been invaluable. I am forever grateful.

A huge thank you to Jo Lal and Beth Bishop. Thank you for your patience, wisdom, and support. This book is better because of your knowledge and guidance.

Tina Manning, thank you for being such an important part of my life—for being my best friend, for laughing with me, and for always supporting me. I'm grateful for you in my life.

Sharon Stone, thank you so much for your continued kindness, care, and generosity and for all of the ways that you have supported me on my journey. And thank you for all of the things you do for our world behind the scenes that most people never see. Thank you!

To my amazing team—Sarah Vogel, Jeff Fenn, Allie Meyer, Cheri Bennett, Brin DeVore, and Brandi Ricole Taylor—thank you so much for being you and for being such an important part of this mission. Thank you for being my team and my friends. As I always say, I could not do this without you. My goal was to have a brilliant, amazing team of kind, loving and smart people who care about the world and the people in it. And each of you is exactly that. Thank you, for being you, for being on this journey with me, and for supporting this mission.

To Brandi Ricole Taylor, a special thank you for being my sounding board and for the countless hours you spent working with me on this book—the late nights and early mornings we spent working on it. I love that it has become your "niece." I love our synergy to work together on projects. I am grateful that we are on this mission together and that you have a big heart and care so much.

Thank you to the pioneers whose work paved the way. Without your research and discoveries, I would likely not have been able to heal myself or bring my work to the world. Thank you for your brilliance, dedication, innovation, and inspiration. Thank you to Fritz-Albert Popp, Florence Scovel Shinn, Louise Hay, Esther Hicks, Alexander Gurwitsch, Sigmund Freud, and so many other brilliant researchers in the areas of psychoneuroimmunology, the placebo, the open-label placebo, MPD/DID, and biophotons. It's because of all of your work that my own healing and work have been possible.

To Veronica Godsend, thank you for being exactly that, a Godsend! I've had so much fun working with you and look forward to working with you on other projects still to come. Thank you for your help in editing and your feedback. Your help has been invaluable, and I appreciate the friendship that developed through this process. You are an incredible being, and you made this process even more enjoyable. I am beyond grateful to you!

Vanessa. No words. Just thank you for being such a wonderful friend throughout this process.

Allison Janse, what would I have done without you? Words are not enough. Thank you for your support, knowledge, insights, edits, and your beautiful heart! You up-leveled the entire book.

Kelly Thompson, I am grateful to you for your brilliant contribution to this book. To say that you up-leveled the entire flow and structure of the book would be an understatement.

The flow is much better, easier, and more accessible because of you! Thank you!

To Thomas Hauck, I am beyond grateful to you! You have been my foundation and my rock. Your role in this entire process has been extremely helpful. Having a full schedule while also writing a book was a challenge, but having you in my corner made everything easier. You have added so much to this project, and I don't know if I could have done this without your help. Thank you for being you!

Jenna Love Shrader, you are such a wonderful editor. Thank you for the loving sweet connection, teamwork, support and accuracy!

To Melanie Bates, your support, insights, and constructive feedback have played a critical role in this process. You are wonderful. Thank you for your heart, your care, and for being you!

Note: If you are reading this wondering why there are so many editors, it is because the original manuscript was almost twice as long as the current edition. So, there was a lengthy process of writing and re-writing, trimming, and re-structuring. And each editor contributed their own magic to help create this book... and I am forever grateful.

To Angela Hartman, thank you for being you! For believing in me and being so helpful in bringing this work to the world. Thank you for being an ally and a friend. I am forever grateful to you!

To Henriett Novak, thank you for being an amazing friend and for all the ways that you have shown up to support me, my work, and this process. I love you and am forever grateful.

Thank you, also, to all those who helped me in other ways on my journey of healing: Rita Brown, Livnat Wilcox, Rodger & Donna Guimond, Lynn Velasquez, Catherine Indovina, Natalia